The Hospitalist Program *Management Guide*

Jeffrey R. Dichter, MD
Leslie E. Cowan, RN, BSN

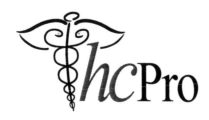

The Hospitalist Program Management Guide is published by HCPro, Inc.

ISBN   1-57839-351-5

Jeffrey R. Dichter, MD, Co-author

Leslie E. Cowan, RN, BSN, Co-author

Erin Callahan, Senior Managing Editor

Rena Mendel, Senior Managing Editor

Julie Pippert, Copyeditor

Jean St. Pierre, Creative Director

Mike Mirabello, Senior Graphic Artist

Matthew Sharpe, Graphic Artist

Layout Artist, Susan Darbyshire

Steve DeGrappo, Cover Designer

Dale Seamans, Executive Editor

Advice given is general. Readers should consult professional counsel for specific, legal, ethical, or clinical questions.

Arrangements can be made for quantity discounts.

For more information, contact:

HCPro, Inc.
P.O. Box 1168
Marblehead, MA 01945
Telephone: 800/650-6787 or 781/639-1872
Fax: 781/639-2982
E-mail: *customerservice@hcpro.com*

Visit HCPro at its World Wide Web sites:
www.hcmarketplace.com, www.hcpro.com,* and *www.msleader.com.

CONTENTS

About the Authors

Jeffrey R. Dichter, MD, FACP

Jeffrey R. Dichter, MD, FACP is a partner of Medical Consultants, PC, a large internal medicine multispecialty group in Muncie, Indiana and is the director of the hospitalist program at Ball Memorial Hospital, also in Muncie. He is currently president of the Society of Hospital Medicine (formerly the National Association of Inpatient Physicians) where he has been a member of its board of directors since February 2000. Dr. Dichter earned his undergraduate degree from the University of California, Berkeley, and graduated from the medical school at the University of Southern California, Los Angeles. He is board certified in both internal and critical care medicine.

Leslie E. Cowan, RN, BSN

Leslie E. Cowan, RN, BSN, is currently the patient placement and resource manager at Ball Memorial Hospital in Muncie, Indiana. Prior to her position at Ball Memorial, Ms. Cowan was the nurse coordinator for the hospitalist group at Medical Consultants, PC, a large multispecialty physician group, also in Muncie, where she was responsible for many of the group's administrative policies. At Medical Consultants, she worked with Dr. Dichter to expand the program from a two-physician group to a seven-physician group with a 24-

hour call schedule. Ms. Cowan is a member of the Society of Hospital Medicine and a member of the National Association of Critical Care Nurses, serving as president of the local chapter from 2001 to 2002. She is a graduate of Ball State University.

Contact information for authors and contributing authors

Leslie E. Cowan, RN, BSN
Patient Placement Nursing Resource Manager
Ball Memorial Hospital
2401 West University Avenue
Muncie, IN 47303

Diane E. Craig, MD, FACP
Assistant Physician-In-Chief
The Permanente Medical Group, Inc.
Clinical Associate Professor of Medicine
Stanford University, School of Medicine
Stanford, CA 94305
diane.craig@kp.org

Jeffrey R. Dichter, MD, FACP
Partner, Medical Consultants, PC
Director, Hospitalist Program
Ball Memorial Hospital
President, Society of Hospital Medicine, (April 2003-April 2004)
2525 University Avenue

Suite 300

Muncie, IN 47303

Jrdichter@iquest.net

Stacy Goldsholl, MD

Medical Director

Catalyst Inpatient Solutions, LLC

Wilmington, NC

stacygoldsholl@msn.com

Mary Jo Gorman, MD, MBA

Chief Medical Officer

IPC-The Hospitalist Company

Office tel.: 800/724-0640

Cell: 888/696-1750

mjgorman@ipcm.com

Patricia M. Gorman, RN, MSM, CPHQ

Director of Case Management

Ball Memorial Hospital

2401 University Avenue

Muncie, IN 47303-3428

Russell Holman, MD

Associate Medical Director, HealthPartners Medical Group & Clinics

Assistant Professor of Medicine, University of Minnesota

Director, Fellowship Program in Hospital Medicine

8100 34th Avenue South

Minneapolis, MN 55440

russell.l.holman@HealthPartners.com

Lee G. Jordan, MD

Executive Vice President,

Chief Medical Officer

Methodist Hospital/Clarian Health (1994-2003)

1801 Senate Boulevard

Indianapolis, IN 46202

ljordan@indy.rr.com

Charleen A. Porter, BS, MA, CPC

Certified Professional Coder

802 E. 206th Street

Sheridan, IN 46069

caporter@insightbb.com

Wayne O. Winney, MHA, CMPE

Chief Operating Officer

Medical Consultants, PC

2525 University Avenue

Suite 300

Muncie, IN 47303

Wowinney@medicalconsultantspc.com

DEDICATION

To my children Claire and Chris, my wonderful children, whose love and support were instrumental to me during this project.
—Leslie Cowan, RN, BSN

To my wife Cathy, and my children Wesleigh, Jay, and Joel. Their patience, love, and support were priceless to me during the preparation of this book.
—Jeff Ditcher, MD

PREFACE

By Jeffrey R. Dichter

In heart and spirit, this book was undertaken to be a "how to" book for hospitalists to build their programs and ensure its continued success. The field of hospital medicine has grown exponentially over the past decade and, remarkably, the growth continues to accelerate.

Over the years, I have had the opportunity to work with hospitalists throughout the country—through the Society of Hospital Medicine (previously National Association of Inpatient Physicians) list serve, at conferences, and when speaking in small group settings. These interactions have made it clear to me that although hospitalists everywhere are building programs, many of these practitioners have little experience or knowledge about much of the administrative, financial, or "systems-know-how" that is necessary to build and maintain an effective program. Therefore, these programs are at risk to fail because of flawed finances, tremendous workloads, or long hours that hospitalist work requires.

Although hospitalist corporations are developing across the country, most programs are still homegrown—built by a relatively small group of local practitioners. A majority of hospitalists are not aware of the program's infrastructure needs, and many of these physicians don't have the time or energy to learn everything they need to know.

These realities fueled our desire to publish a book that discussed all the issues hospitalists must address to successfully practice, and provided references for information that did not fit in the book to guide hospitalists' research. We aimed to provide hospitalists with the tools to build and maintain great hospitalist programs.

Section one of this book focuses on the needs of customers. Hospitalists who know who their customers are and what their needs are, have the best chance of building successful programs. Rusty Holman, who authored Chapter 1, was instrumental in building a large hospitalist program at Health Partners in Minneapolis, MN, and is truly expert at understanding the needs of referring physicians. Lee Jordan, executive vice president at Methodist Hospital in Indianapolis, IN, —author of Chapter 2—worked with the organization's hospitalist programs and other physician-based groups. Jordan believes that hospitalist programs and hospitals are most successful when their relationship is built on understanding and good faith. Because most programs are at least partially underwritten by hospitals, the information in this chapter may be among the most important in this book. Diane Craig, author of Chapter 3, has extensive experience with Kaiser Permanente of Northern California, and is a staunch, passionate patient advocate,

Section two focuses on the hospitalist program's needs. The key issues for any program revolve around communication, systems of care, resource security, efficiency and quality data, development of young hospitalists, finances, and coding. The expert contributors in this section include Stacy Goldscholl, Pat Gorman, MaryJo Gorman, Wayne Winney, Charlene Porter, and Leslie Cowan. Each of these professionals has a broad practical knowledge of their field of expertise, and an ability to communicate it effectively.

I also contributed to section two of this book. I acquired much of my understanding of hospital medicine by accepting the privilege of leadership positions at the Society of Hospital Medicine (SHM). I am grateful for the opportunity to serve in these positions and to work with outstanding professionals who are members of SHM—some of whom also contributed to this book. I encourage all hospitalists to look for other SHM resources.

Lastly, I would like to thank all of you—the practicing hospitalists throughout the country. I draw inspiration and motivation from my interactions with you all.

Hospitalist Program Stakeholders: Primary and Specialty Care Physicians

Russell Holman, MD

The hospitalist movement in the United States has grown tremendously since the late 1990s—a trend that will likely characterize the delivery of inpatient care for years to come. Driving this movement is the need to reduce health care costs and enhance acute care skills for managing complex patients, as well as hospitals' desire to advance quality and safety through physician champions. But perhaps the most prevalent and controversial factor contributing to the growth of hospitalist programs is primary and specialty physicians' desire to implement such programs.

Although this chapter will focus on the value that other physicians place on the services provided by hospitalists, it is important to first review some of the concerns primary and specialty physicians have traditionally expressed about unconditionally welcoming hospitalist programs into the health care system. In early hospitalist programs, primary and specialty care physicians cited several potential drawbacks to unconditional welcome/acceptance of a hospitalist.

For example, primary care physicians (PCPs) were concerned that hospitalist programs would result in decreased patient-service revenue and acute care clinical skills, loss of direct patient care continuity, increased outpatient acuity, and complexity due to shorter lengths of stay, decreased patient acceptance, and loss of clinical autonomy.

Specialty care physicians were also hesitant to accept hospitalists. These physicians were worried that implementing a hospitalist program would result in fewer formal consultation requests and delayed consultation requests. In addition, specialists were concerned about hospitalists' scope of clinical practices, and their potential negative effect on the emergency department (ED). Further, the introduction of hospitalists made medical academics concerned about that scope of educational and research practices

Because of the numerous concerns raised by the introduction of hospitalists, careful planning and conscientious measurement of results is critical to provide feedback and reassurance to key stakeholders.

Cultural variables

Many of the previously mentioned issues are highly variable and determined by the practice location. The culture and values of a hospital, medical staff, and related medical groups are diverse and do not necessarily follow a predictable pattern according to institution type (e.g., major academic, community non-teaching, etc.), hospital size, geographic location, payer mix, or specialty training (e.g., orthopedic surgery, family medicine, cardiology, etc.).

Each practice setting requires an independent and comprehensive assessment of the culture, values, and strategic priorities to determine the proposed hospitalist program's suitability and scope. Remember that the organization must also assess whether it has considered all relevant issues when expanding or changing the scope of an existing hospitalist group.

To explore your local culture and values, ask specialty and primary care colleagues what they believe the hospitalist's role is in the health care system. By approaching the topic from this perspective, a sense of collaboration is created with stakeholders in developing or modifying the hospitalist program. Furthermore, it illustrates an understanding of the complex interdependence within the delivery system by underscoring the relativity of each component to the whole. In other words, it is very different for a group of potential hospitalists to sit in a room and plan their practice parameters v. an open-ended discussion with PCPs, hospital administrators, and surgical specialists.

Consider, for example, the experience of a hospital that included clinic-based generalist physicians. The hospitalist group entered the conversation with the assumption that they would serve as patients' PCPs in the hospital, coordinating care with all other parties and then returning care to the clinic physician when patients were transitioned out of the inpatient setting. However, once the organization's culture was fully examined—its values openly discussed and patients' needs considered above all—it reached a subtly different conclusion. In the revised system, the hospitalist serves as a consultant to the PCP during the inpatient stay, coordinates care, and returns direct patient care responsibility once the hospitalization has ended. This new perspective, with emphasis on PCPs' sense of ownership of patients throughout the care continuum has strong implications for preservation of longitudinal care planning, PCPs' social visits in the hospital, and communication expectations among providers.

General principles

Now that the fundamental questions of program purpose and relativity have been addressed, it's time to discuss a framework for ensuring the value of the hospitalist program. A successful hospitalist program should be built on six generally principles, all of which are relevant to primary and specialty concerns. Through methodical consideration of these principles, a blueprint for interactions with other stakeholders is devised.

The six general principles are as follows:

1. Value

A value equation seen repeatedly in health care and other industries is a valid means by which to judge various products or services. It is as follows:

$$\text{Value} = \frac{\text{Quality x Satisfaction}}{\text{Cost}}$$

This equation illustrates the notion that products and services are most often deemed valuable, or to add value, if they are high in quality, satisfying, and cost effective. The denominator usually refers to the sponsor's financial commitment, but may also include indirect monetary costs, political "capital," time, educational needs, emotional investment, facilities, or other support services. Satisfaction is largely self-explanatory and, in the context of this chapter, refers to the satisfaction of other physician stakeholders.

2. Quality

Quality assessment in health care can best be described by the six characteristics outlined in the 2001 Institute of Medicine Report *Crossing the Quality Chasm.*

For example, starting with safety as a system property, quality naturally demands that avoidable errors be dramatically reduced or eliminated. Timely care eliminates unnecessary waiting and ensures ready access to services. The system should also be effective, delivering care that is evidence-based and known to be beneficial while simultaneously withholding unhelpful or harmful interventions. Efficient care reduces waste, rework, and duplication. A system that provides care to all patients regardless of race, gender, religious, or socioeconomic status is deemed equitable. Perhaps most importantly is the element of patient-centeredness: The system must reflect preferences and priorities based on the individual values and goals of the patient and must include him or her in care planning and decisions.

3. Alignment

Alignment is a natural consequence of determining purpose and relativity. It is rare for a hospitalist program to single-handedly alter the strategic course of a medical group or organization. Rather, it may be an important step in aligning care and services according to an existing strategic plan. Aligning program design with a common vision held by key stakeholders will help to ensure success.

4. Partnership

If alignment implies compliance with a broader system values, partnership is the means by which compliance translates into relationships. Hospitalists and primary/specialty care physicians must establish a mutual understanding regarding the primary and specialty care physicians' influence on program development and operations. Inviting other physicians to design, recruit for, provide feedback to, and collaborate with hospitalists will yield a deliberate and well-constructed hospitalist program.

5. Professionalism

Professionalism is frequently discussed in medical literature. Therefore, this book will not attempt to reproduce a comprehensive definition or to describe the current state of medical professionalism. However, it is imperative that hospitalist programs incorporate the tenets of professionalism, including the application of specialized knowledge and commitment to service.

There are two commonly cited phenomena within professionalism that deserve special attention. First is the evolution of hospital medicine, which may be seen as a threat to the autonomy of traditional specialties and subspecialties and may result in a defensive stance that can undermine successful collaboration. Second, medical socialization—especially during training—may engender intraprofessional disrespect through informal means, also called the "hidden curriculum" in medical education. Awareness of these two phenomena will allow each hospitalist program to define the parameters of optimal professionalism and avoid pitfalls of overlooking the virtues of effective collaboration and appropriate medical socialization.

6. Ambiguity

Let's face it: There are few certainties in the future of hospital medicine. This is no surprise given the enormous variety of existing hospitalist programs—all differ in purpose, design, management, goals, staffing, settings, training, scope of practice, and measures of success.

The effects of ambiguity are seen in organizations around the country. For example, in larger organizations, particularly academic institutions, there is much debate over where to "house" a hospitalist program—within the general internal medicine or general pediatrics department, the primary care division, or the medical specialties? Create a new department of hospital medicine?

Furthermore, the absence of specific training requirements or certification, coupled with hospital privileging and credentialing issues, creates further uncertainty about the development and operations of a hospitalist program. By directly and openly confronting ambiguity within one's own local environment, questions can be addressed, partnerships strengthened, and concerns alleviated.

Hospitalists' value to primary care

From the PCPs' perspective, the value equation is primarily driven by the factors in the numerator: quality and satisfaction. Although PCPs do keep an eye on associated costs, it is less of a concern. PCPs commonly measure the value of a hospitalist service based on the following factors:

- **Effective communication**

  There is no greater value in the eyes of a PCP than maintaining effective communication on clinical matters. A hospitalist's communication with PCPs may affect all elements of the value equation—perceived higher quality of care, higher PCP satisfaction, and lower costs in the form of less duplication of effort. One of the most vulnerable moments for patients is the transition to and from the hospital setting—moments often accompanied by insufficient information transfer during the handoff. Without compensating for this with formalized expectations of communication, quality of care is at risk. For example, safety (e.g., inappropriate medications or doses administered), efficiency (e.g., duplication of effort), and timeliness (e.g., delays in evaluation and management) can be negatively affected if transition of care is not addressed.

PCP satisfaction is at stake not only for reasons of quality, but also for continuity of care and preservation of long-term patient/family relationships. Consider the following scenario:

Dr. Smith, a PCP, is shopping in the grocery store and is approached by Mrs. Jones, the wife of Dr. Smith's patient for 13 years. Mrs. Jones inquires as to whether anything more could have been done for her husband—did she do the right thing "signing those papers"? Dr. Smith, politely asking the circumstances surrounding her inquiry, learns of Mr. Jones' inpatient death nearly two weeks earlier and is faced with explaining his ignorance to a puzzled and distraught family member.

• **Education**

Communication need not be looked at as a mechanical, rote task of information transfer. The most progressive hospitalist groups—those that successfully partner with PCP colleagues—view communication as the means to provide education. The hospital setting is often where complex management decisions are made, high technology procedures are used, and cutting-edge therapies are implemented. These activities require more than a passive mention to the accepting PCP. They require elaboration on how and why they were selected, the potential benefits and complications, the rationale in the context of the patient's longitudinal plan of care, and the recommended follow up and treatment duration.

Education of PCPs may also take the form of more traditional methods for clinic-based physicians who wish to maintain their hospital knowledge and skills. Continuing medical education (CME) programs, dedicated mentorship, journal clubs, grand rounds, newsletters, and e-mail supporting the professional interests of PCPs are highly valuable educational tools.

- **Focus of practice**
  Decreasing complexity in the PCP's professional scope may be highly desirable and significantly enhance work satisfaction. Reducing or eliminating daytime, weekend, holiday, and night hospital responsibilities enables the PCP to pay closer attention to routine clinic systems and patients. The PCP and clinical support staff's work schedules may become more predictable with the introduction of hospitalists.

  Without inpatient care demands, the PCP can also participate in focused CME programs to improve essential ambulatory skills, including medical orthopedics or alternative medicine. In short, a PCP's opportunity to give up hospital practice might prove to be a valuable quality of a hospitalist program.

- **Access**

  Patients appreciate the ability to conveniently schedule an appointment with their PCPs. The patient's ability to do so translates both directly and indirectly into PCP satisfaction in the form of reduced patient complaints, reduced patient attrition from clinic panels, and potential strengthening of the PCP-patient relationship by fewer "diverts" to other clinic-practice colleagues. A hospitalist program that substantially improves outpatient-clinic access adds value to both the PCP and the community.

- **Unassigned patients**

  Helping PCPs focus on their outpatient practice alleviates PCP liability for unassigned patients admitted to the hospital. The responsibility for unassigned patients, which is commonly distributed across the hospital medical staff, often disrupts clinic schedules and outpatient access. Unassigned patients may also have a less favorable payer mix, which can lead to decreased patient service revenues for a PCP's practice—another undesirable outcome of this obligation.

- **Revenues**

  There are three places that a hospitalist program may positively affect PCP revenues. First, as mentioned above, is the assumption of unassigned patient call. Second, the elimination of travel time to and from the hospital may translate directly into increased patient encounters at the clinic. Finally, because of the unpredictable nature of inpatient work volumes, increased clinical productivity in the office may be more lucrative and reliable.

• **Mentorship**

Hybrid models of inpatient care—those that employ both hospitalists and clinic-based physicians to provide direct clinical services—lend themselves to clinical mentorship by hospitalists. A PCP whose main professional focus is on ambulatory medicine will value working along side hospitalists in the acute setting. A formally or informally structured mentorship program in which the hospitalist provides the PCP with guidance regarding clinical problem-solving, management, or hospital systems of care can enhance PCP satisfaction, efficiency, and ensure quality of care.

• **Links with subspecialists**

The hospital has traditionally been a venue where PCPs and subspecialty physicians interact developing collegial relationships and discussing patient care issues. These interactions form the basis for both referral patterns and personal friendships. As PCPs remove themselves from this professional socialization, reliance on hospitalists to bridge those interactions and relationships are increasingly important. The hospitalist's value to a PCP will come in the form of linking physicians who are geographically separated through effective communication and education.

• **Consulting roles**

Hospitalists often consider their scope of practice to extend beyond the direct care of medical or pediatric inpatients to include medical consultation practices. PCPs may view the on-site presence of hospitalists as a significant benefit to patients who receive surgical, psychiatric, or other specialty services. Whether taking the form of prompt preoperative assessments, dedicated surgical comanagement systems, or problem-specific consultations, PCP's will appreciate the hospitalists' generalist approach to their patients. Furthermore, hospitalists can offer PCPs a second opinion for patients with clinical problems that were either elusive or refractory in the ambulatory setting.

- **Palliative care**

  The medical community is increasing awareness of the need to improve end-of-life care. In few other settings is this need more acutely warranted than in the institutional setting. This topic is strongly emphasized in hospitalists' professional education and provides an opportunity to devise effective inpatient models of care. Hospitalists who demonstrate commitment to these activities will be favorably regarded by their PCP colleagues.

Hospitalists' value to specialty care

Like PCPs, specialty care physicians commonly measure the value of a hospitalist service based on the following factors, which relate to quality and satisfaction:

- **Effective communication**

  Most of the key concepts of this factor are outlined above. Communication serves as the linchpin for all other value elements.

- **Education**

  The generalist approach taken by hospitalists may serve as a useful method of educating specialty care physicians on patient care issues outside their respective expertise.

- **Access**

  Hospitalists' ability to improve patient flow may enhance the organization's capacity to accommodate specialty patients. Increasing the number of available beds for elective and emergent cases enables specialty care physicians to focus their efforts on preferred hospital sites.

- **Intensive care unit (ICU) interface**

  Defining in advance those patients assigned to a hospitalist or an intensivist may alleviate the potential tension between these groups. This exercise can also provide the basis for further discussion regarding consultation practices and the transition when an ICU patient under the care of an intensivist is ready to move to a general care bed.

- **Surgical-hospitalist comanagement**

  Many hospitals, both academic and community, have implemented hospitalists models that encourage surgical-hospitalist comanagement. This model can enhance surgical specialists' satisfaction, including orthopedics, urology, otolaryngology, and neurosurgery.

  Comanagement alleviates physicians' discomfort with problems outside the range of their expertise, speeds up pre- and perioperative assessment, reduces post-surgical complications, enhances coordination of care, ensures guideline compliance, decreases the time spent on the ward, and increases the time devoted to performing surgery. Further, comanagement can increase surgical volume, which leads to increased patient service revenues.

- **Professional focus**

  Specialty care physicians are in short supply in some organizations. Hospitalists who serve as the attending physician of record and coordinate the care of specialty patients allow the specialty care physician to focus on consultative efforts, procedural interventions, outreach practices, and other means of leveraging their specialized knowledge. In this regard, hospitalist practices may increase the efficiency of specialty practices.

- **Consultation request**

  Specialty care physicians can best provide needed services when requests for their support are timely and precise. Specialists often contend that their early involvement in complex cases will likely lead to improved patient outcomes. Therefore, by clearly specifying the problem to be addressed and by communicating requests directly to the consultant, hospitalists help equip specialty care physicians to render a high-quality consultative response.

- **Acceptance of referrals**

  Specialty care physicians who perform outreach activities or who are in short supply of staff may not have a consistent on-site presence at the hospital. Hospitalists enhance value by accepting inpatient referrals and transfers and seamlessly coordinating care for these patients in the specialty care physician's temporary absence.

- **ED**

  Hospitalists who appropriately execute ED services enhance satisfaction and efficiency of emergency care providers. When supported by hospitalist programs, the following services may benefit emergency physicians and their departments:

  - Facilitation of patient transitions from ED to inpatient bed, with emphasis on prompt communication and initiation of care protocols

  - Triage of patients to appropriate levels of care within the hospital (e.g., ICU v. telemetry)

  - Risk-sharing in making collaborative decisions

  - Acceptance of transfers from outside hospitals and facilitation of direct admission transfers when able (previously, the ED physician may have been the only point of facility contact for the hospital)

  - Timely performance of medical or pediatric consultation as a value-added service, as opposed to having only phone access to a clinic-based physician

- Assumption of management responsibilities of patients within an observation unit

- Solution to the unassigned patient issue, which traditionally falls to the ED to engage the hospital medical staff with variable success and enthusiasm

Value-based program development

Building a hospitalist program committed to rendering value to key stakeholders requires assimilating the six general principles described earlier into a logical and sequential approach. In essence, organizations can follow a model for creating a hospitalist program that improves quality and satisfaction while lowering cost.

Many organizations fail to create an organized, comprehensive, value-based long-term plan when developing a new hospitalists program. Focusing on short-term needs, internal political pressures, timeline pressures, or having a narrow scope of stakeholder engagement will betray the best intentions of the program. Remember: An aspiring program that has a three-month development period preceding implementation and is fully aligned with the hospital administration's priorities will fail, partially or completely, if partnership with specialty and primary care has not been adequately secured.

What follows is a 12-step process to ensure that value is a driving force in program development. Each step includes practical aspects founded in well-established concepts of management, performance improvement, and collaboration. Although many of the steps appear to occur in a linear fashion, some must take place concurrently, or directly loop back to earlier steps.

Step 1: Establish program purpose, values, and goals

As discussed earlier in this chapter, PCPs and specialty care physicians must be included in the development of the hospitalist program to ensure a culture of teamwork through alignment, partnership, professionalism, and specificity.

Step 2: Define hospitalists' roles and responsibilities

This step leads to the formation of a job description and helps set very clear expectations for what it means to be a valued contributor the hospitalist program's success. Job descriptions should make clear how hospitalists should interact with PCPs and specialty care physicians.

Step 3: Determine the organizational structure

Reporting structures, departmental allocations, and medical staff structures should be addressed early in the development process. Although in some settings these decisions may be straightforward, in others it may be politically charged and require prudent mediation. This step reduces ambiguity and allows for a tangible reference point for other members of a medical group or hospital medical staff.

Step 4: Recruit the right people

Using program goals and values as your guide, recruit hospitalists based on their ability to help achieve program success. Having the right people on board is arguably the most important factor in animating the program's purpose and creating a high-performance team.

Step 5: Identify key stakeholders

This step closely follows or accompanies the process of setting clear expectations. Hospitalists need to know what is expected of them, how they should interact with other practitioners and hospital personnel, and who their "customers" are.

Step 6: Measure performance

Measurement should be both formal (e.g., referring physician satisfaction surveys) and informal. For example, nurses, PCPs, and specialty colleagues should be surveyed regarding interactions with hospitalists.

Step 7: Provide feedback

The art and science of delivering performance feedback is beyond the scope of this chapter. However, keep in mind that the key elements of effective feedback include timeliness and specificity. Feedback should be consistently provided to hospitalists, PCPs, and specialty care providers to encourage performance improvement and reinforce positive practices.

Step 8: Make adaptations

Once measurement has led to feedback, adaptations in program structure, operations, expectations, interactions, and/or methods may be made to render greater value to stakeholders.

Step 9: Align incentives

In many medical groups, PCP satisfaction regarding communication and quality of care account for a portion of hospitalists' variable compensation. However, incentives need not be financial. Consider the power of non-monetary rewards such as public recognition and incremental leadership responsibilities.

Step 10: Manage results

A high-performance program must include effective mechanisms to celebrate success as well as to correct marginal or egregious behavior.

Step 11: Continuously assess expectations

Expectations for the hospitalist program should be constantly assessed during performance evaluations, group meetings, interactions with PCP and specialty care provider leaders. After implementing the previous 10 steps, the organization can reaffirm existing expectations and introduce new expectations of performance.

Step 12: Watch for pitfalls

There are too many factors that can potentially undermine program success to be listed here. However, an astute hospitalist program leader will strive to anticipate and proactively solve problems.

Properly conceived and implemented hospitalist programs bring value to primary and specialty care physicians. When designing such a model of care, organizations must first understand the factors of quality, satisfaction, and cost and their relative importance in determining value. A hospitalist program devised through careful consideration and discussion of its purpose and value members of the health care system will have a strong foundation. This foundation will allow the hospitalist group to tackle the operational challenges that may arise. Values direct the group's recruitment strategies, set performance goals, and determine incentives. Moreover, values defined in partnership with specialty and primary care stakeholders will ease the program's integration into the local culture and set the ethical standards for the shared care of patients.

References

Cohn, SL. "The role of the medical consultant," *Med Clin N Am,* 2003; 87:1-6.

Frey, J. "The clinical philosophy of family medicine." *American Journal of Medicine,* 1998; 104:327–329.

Institute of Medicine. *Crossing the Quality Chasm: A New Health System for the 21st Century.* National Academy Press, 2001.

Papadakis, MA. "Do as I say, not as I do," *American Journal of Medicine,* 1998; 104:605–606.

Stern, DT. "Practicing what we preach? An analysis of the curriculum of values in medical education," *American Journal of Medicine,* 1998; 104:569–575.

Stoeckle JD, LJ Ronan, LL Emanuel, Ehrlich CM. "A manual on manners and courtesies for the shared care of patients," *Journal of Clinical Ethics,* 1997;8(1):22–33.

Wortmann, RL. "The clinical philosophy of internal medicine," *American Journal of Medicine,* 1998; 104:323–326.

HOSPITALISTS:
THE HOSPITAL PERSPECTIVE

LEE G. JORDAN, MD

The history of hospital-physician relationships is long and diverse. These relationships can be based on simple understandings, guided by carefully constructed contracts, or managed through employment agreements. Relationships between physicians and hospitals are ideally based on mutual trust and shared goals, but all too often they are shaped by physicians' and hospitals' fear of one another. In today's complicated medical environment, it's important to establish effective relationships between physicians and hospitals that are founded on mutually understood and measurable goals.

Hospitals' increasing need for hospitalists offers an opportunity to construct effective relationships between hospitals and physicians. These relationships improve patient care outcomes, meet hospital and physician business needs, and increase patient satisfaction.

In this chapter, we will explore how hospitals and physicians can establish an effective relationship to improve patient care and secure fiscal health. Hospitalists can play an important role in establishing such relationships. The growth of hospitalist programs should improve hospitals' and physicians' understanding of one another's responsibilities, challenges, and goals.

The effectiveness equation

Hospitals are increasingly relying on and investing in hospitalists. However, the nature and scale of such investments vary considerably from hospital to hospital. In addition, hospitals' confidence in these investments varies.

Hospitals and physicians may find the following equation, which expresses both the investment and the value of hospitalists, useful in overcoming hesitations about relying on these practitioners. Very simply put, the hospital would like to say:

$$\textbf{Effectiveness} \geq \textbf{Investment}$$

In this chapter, we will discuss how hospitals define effectiveness and investments. Keep in mind, if hospitals and physicians work together to construct this equation and faithfully follow it, the hospital environment will improve for hospitalists, primary care physicians (PCPs), and specialists.

Figure 2.1 illustrates the elements of the effectiveness equation and the categories we will explore in this chapter. It's important that hospital leaders and hospitalists understand the effectiveness side of the equation. This understanding is essential to clarify goals before the controversial subjects of finances and control are discussed.

Common barriers to change

Hospital administrators and physicians must first tackle a few common challenges before they can successfully measure effectiveness.

The first of these is establishing the *validity of data*. Hospital systems are often inaccurate and incomplete. Until decision support systems and computerized medical information systems evolve, hospitals and physicians are forced to make the best use of the information available.

Hospital decision support systems must contain diagnosis, complication, and outcomes data. Analysis of this information can identify improvement opportunities and allow hospitals to track such improvements.

To make the best use of the information contained in decision support systems, hospitalists must understand how the systems work and develop a relationship with hospital personnel who manage it. The hospital's financial department often controls these systems, and too often there is little communication between the department and physicians. However, it is important that the information is effectively delivered to hospitalists or that hospitalists have the ability to create their own queries and reports. If hospitalists can use this information to improve the care, they will gain considerable credibility with the medical staff.

Effective electronic medical records (EMR) provide numerous opportunities to improve inpatient care and outcome measurement. Unfortunately, many EMRs are far from perfect, which often results in a skeptical and defensive medical staff. Hospitalists should partner with key medical staff members to improve the effectiveness of the organization's EMRs and increase the medical staff's acceptance of such systems. If the hospital and its consultants lead this project, the medical staff may consider the system to be ineffective. Hospitalists' wide scope of care makes them well equipped to take the lead in this arena.

The second obstacle relates to *cause and effect*. The effectiveness of a hospital's investment is affected by multiple factors. Therefore, it is often difficult to assert that the hospitalist program is solely responsible for the improvement or decline of an investment's effectiveness. However, it is possible to use carefully selected measures to determine the positive effect of implementing a hospitalist program.

It is therefore critical for hospitalists to familiarize themselves with other organizational activities and variables to correctly assess their program's ability to enact positive change.

For example, hospitalists may work closely with the medical and nursing staff to develop and implement the hospital's diabetes-care protocol. The hospitalists partner with other practitioners to design patient profiles, deliver education, administer insulin, and provide clinical follow-up. Although the protocol may be effective, it will be difficult to measure its impact immediately. In addition, other factors—new medical staff members or nurse educators—may contribute to reducing diabetes patients' lengths of stay and blood sugar outcomes. Because of the complexity of inpatient care and the difficulty conducting data analysis, it is nearly impossible to examine each factor separately. Hospitalists should assume a leadership position when implementing such programs and carefully monitor outcomes. However, hospitalists must acknowledge the complexity of cause and effect and avoid claiming sole credit for improvements.

Define effectiveness

There are several ways a hospital measures its return on investments. Medical and business literature, as well as unpublished practical experience, provides numerous examples of how to measure the effectiveness of investments.

Take a look at the following sample framework organizations can use to measure the benefits/return on investment of its hospitalist program:

1. Patient flow
2. Fixed and variable cost item improvements
3. Quality of care and patient safety

4. Patient satisfaction

5. Physician satisfaction

6. Nursing satisfaction

7. Physician productivity

Patient flow

Hospitals are motivated to improve patient flow because reimbursement con-tracts are often driven by a fixed-payment per diagnosis or case. Therefore, a hospital expends less cost per fixed-reimbursement when a patient efficiently moves through the facility. Keep in mind that the prevalence of this particu-lar reimbursement scheme differs by market, but it does apply to most large institutions.

Patient-flow concerns also arise when hospitals attempt to increase their capacity to provide care in profitable specialties such as cardiovascular surgery, orthopedics, and neurosurgery.

Geriatric patients and patients who require complex surgery typically slow down a hospital's patient flow. Hospitalists can assist the hospital by provid-ing care to these patients, allowing the organization to increase its profitabili-ty and satisfy both the medical staff and patient's demands for shorter wait times.

Patient flow is a challenge for many organizations. A hospitalist program can-not resolve all of the hospital's patient-flow issues, but it can improve patient flow by focusing on the following factors:

- **Lengths of stay**

  Most hospital decision support systems contain extensive length of stay data. This information can be compared to national and regional data to identify improvement opportunities.

  Once the hospitalist identifies the hospital's improvement needs, he or she should consult published studies that discuss how length of stay can be shortened without negatively affecting quality of care. The hospitalists can then target the areas of the hospital in which they practice and present the organization with a clear before-and-after picture that clearly shows how the hospitalist program has reduced patients' lengths of stay.

  Further, many hospital decision support systems collect information about "delay days" This information can also identify improvement opportunities. Therefore, hospitalists must establish a cooperative relationship with hospital personnel who control these systems. (See Chapter 7 for more information about data needs and information assessment.)

- **Emergency department (ED) flow**

  EDs often struggle to rapidly collect the patient's disposition, find an appropriate physician to treat the patient, and move the patient to the patient care unit for treatment. Although a hospitalists' involvement in the ED may not directly transfer to hospital savings, it can reduce delays in the overall care process. Hospitalist programs should work with ED leadership and medical staff to identify such opportunities.

Hospitalists' ED duties vary depending on hospital staffing, availability of PCPs and specialists, and the number of hospitalists. Hospitalists and the medical staff should consider these variables when determining the hospitalists' availability (e.g., 24-seven, nighttime) and range of services (e.g., evaluation, admission, ongoing care, and discharge planning). Although it can be helpful to know how other organizations have designed their hospitalist programs, solutions must be organization-specific. Hospitals should work with medical staff members and hospitalists to develop a local solution.

- **Critical care observation cases**
  Critical care patients in the intensive care unit (ICU) often do not receive needed critical care treatment, but rather are simply observed. Although many cases that fall into this observation-only category benefit from ICU care, some may be handled with little or no ICU care.

  Hospitalists can address this problem by increasing the medical staff's confidence in off-site ICU care facilities, creating appropriate "step down" areas, and clarifying the responsibilities of caregivers from outside of the ICU to critical care physicians. Many hospitalists work with critical care staff to reduce ICU admissions and appropriately transfer patients out of the unit. The hospital supports such partnerships because of reimbursement patterns and the high cost of ICU treatment. Beyond fiscal concerns, a partnership between hospitalists and critical care physicians can improve the quality of patient care by increasing the availability of critical care resources

The key players in the patient-flow process (e.g., ED and operating room [OR] staff, nursing, critical care physicians, large practices, and hospitalists) need a process map by which to evaluate the data and variables. A process map guides the key players to develop solutions that allow hospitalists to assume care for specific patient groups. Therefore, hospitalists and critical care physicians should work together to create a process map and gather relevant data. The two groups should then gather support from the nursing, operations, medical, and ED staff.

- **OR flow**

  Hospitalists can improve OR flow by improving the outflow of patients in the intensive and critical care units. If critical care units and medical surgical units are full, the hospital may need to cancel or delay OR cases, which results in lost revenue and frustrated surgeons.

  Hospitalists and key surgical staff should discuss the hospital's policies and procedures that guide preoperative evaluation, admission, inpatient care, and discharge planning. Not all surgeons think alike, but many will welcome the opportunity to partner with hospitalists to make their hospital practice more efficient and improve patient outcomes. As these processes are clarified, the hospitalists and surgeons can turn to the hospital to help with resource needs, such as space for a preoperative clinic.

- **Patient discharge**

  Many patient-flow studies identify discharge time as an opportunity. Hospitals often discharge patients in the afternoon. Therefore, hospitalists should examine the organization's existing discharge practices and partner with nursing and medical staff to discharge more patients in the morning—improving lengths of stay and delay data.

• **Readmission**

Patients are readmitted to the hospital for many reasons. These readmissions cost hospitals money, especially when they involve Medicare or Medicaid patients. Many insurers, including the Center for Medicare & Medicaid Services, will not pay hospitals for readmissions. Therefore, readmissions add to the hospital's cost, inhibiting personnel or facility upgrades.

Hospitalists should work with the hospital medical staff to target key populations and improve the discharge process—including instruction and follow-up—and decrease readmission rates.

Organizations often fail to successfully address patient flow challenges because they traditionally turn to physicians for help—physicians who often focus solely on their department, practice, or specialty's interests. Hospitalists are well-positioned to help hospitals improve patient flow and significantly increase the organization's efficiency and quality.

Many institutions fail to assign accountability for patient flow. It's time for hospitals to follow the lead of power plants that focus on energy distribution and airports that track airline arrivals and departures. Hospitalist program leaders should partner with hospital, medical staff, and nursing leaders to undertake "inpatient engineering." See **Figure 2.2** for additional information about successful engineering of the acute care process.

Fixed and variable cost items

Fixed and variable cost items include blood products, drugs, and medical devices. Hospitalists can help hospitals standardize these items to save money. For example, an organization that uses two antibiotics in one class instead of five is in a better position to negotiate with the pharmaceutical company for lower unit prices. Hospitalists should work with the organization's pharmacist to identify such opportunities and join the hospital's pharmacy and therapeutics committee.

Staffing is another important cost that hospitalists can influence. Hospitalists can partner with nursing and medical staff leaders to determine appropriate clinical staffing levels. A large patient care engineering project conducted by hospitalists in conjunction with other organizational leaders will often identify additional improvement opportunities.

For example, a patient-care engineering project that focuses on a specific department (e.g., ED, OR, or ICU) may lead to a more efficient use of nursing staff or identify a need for additional staff.

Quality of care and patient safety

Hospitalists have numerous opportunities to improve the quality and safety of patient care, such as standardizing the treatment of pneumonia patients and diabetics and tracking complication and mortality rates. Remember that these activities should be aligned with hospital-wide quality programs approved by the medical staff and board of directors. Turn to **Figure 2.3** to review the Institute of Medicine's 20 quality priorities, which the organization outlined in January 2003. **Figure 2.4** provides a few examples of how hospitalists can address these priorities.

In addition, hospitalists and the medical staff should set specific quality goals (e.g., improving the timeliness of antibiotics administration for pneumonia patients). Hospitalists should track the affect of improvement activities and include that data in their effectiveness report.

Hospitalists should also be involved in the development of the hospital's computerized medical information systems, as well as the processes these systems aim to improve (e.g., medication ordering and delivery). Nearly every hospital has a process for developing an EMR—though some organizations may only be in the discussion phase of the project. Hospitalists should take the following steps to contribute to the development of an EMR:

1. Understand the organization's existing process

2. Expand knowledge of medical informatics

3. Seek out and establish good relations with medical staff currently involved with the project

Patient satisfaction

Some medical experts are concerned that patients will not accept hospitalists. However, current medical literature, experience, and studies indicate that patients do accept hospitalists when the hospitalist program is managed effectively and staffed by caring practitioners.

As patients continue to recognize hospitalists' positive effect on patient care —including the ability to quickly address a patient's question or problem during the hours that the attending physician is unavailable—the acceptance of these new practitioners will increase. Increased patient satisfaction is yet another indication of hospitalists' effectiveness.

Most hospitals have a patient-satisfaction tracking system. But because these systems vary from hospital to hospital, each organization's ability to measure hospitalists' effect on patient satisfaction will also vary. However, all organizations that want to measure hospitalists' effect on patient satisfaction must determine how to use a subset of this data. Therefore, hospitals may find it easier to design a new system to evaluate patient satisfaction in regard to the hospitalist program.

Hospitalists should track improvements in patient satisfaction rates and present evidence of these improvements to hospital leadership. Keep in mind that patient satisfaction is affected by numerous factors—many of which fall outside the purview of the hospitalist program. However, it is important for hospitals to discuss patient satisfaction with the organization's leaders and use this information to identify opportunities for improvement.

Many private vendors that provide patient satisfaction data to hospitals can collect information that is specific to a patient care unit or patient type. Hospitalists should review this data with the nursing and medical staff periodically and suggest improvements. Depending on their scope of care, hospitalists may be directly involved in implementing changes that will increase patient satisfaction.

Physician satisfaction

Hospitals are more likely to formally evaluate patient satisfaction than physician satisfaction. However, physician satisfaction is a priority for hospital leaders and governing boards. Hospital leaders and board members want objective evaluations that point the way to improvements. Hospitals are currently at different stages in regard to physician satisfaction evaluations. However, whether the facility has just implemented a physician-satisfaction measurement program or has just started discussing such a program, hospitalists can help. The organization's hospitalists should find out where in this the process the institution is and develop a strategy of engagement and partnership.

Hospitalists can enhance primary care and subspecialty physician satisfaction in regard to lifestyle and business interests. It's important that hospitalists understand how to measure their impact on physician satisfaction, present this information to the hospital, and align themselves with hospital leaders working on the organization's physician satisfaction program.

Hospitalists should develop a strategy and timeline for partnering with the key practice groups working at the hospital to understand the needs of the physicians in each group. Studying the strengths and weaknesses of each practice will allow hospitalists to develop a plan to effectively improve physician satisfaction. This is an ambitious and ongoing project.

Some hospitals employ physician leaders to act as liaisons between the organization and group practices. Hospitalists should partner with such leaders rather than taking on this task alone.

Nursing satisfaction

The availability of knowledgeable hospitalists can significantly increase nurse satisfaction. Acute care is a series of questions and decisions. In routine cases, these questions and answers are managed by an accepted protocol. However, many cases are not routine. Hospitalists can help nurses make decisions and take immediate action when faced with challenging cases.

The nursing and medical staff often require the advice of experts when revising old protocols and developing new guidelines. Hospitalists can improve nurse satisfaction by getting involved in this process.

Hospitalists often receive high marks from nurses because they are consistently available to answer questions and discuss patient care. On a more prospective basis, hospitalists can identify and help design specific "care engineering" opportunities.

In addition, because hospitalists provide timely patient care and implement improved protocols and pathways, the nursing staff can eventually make staffing changes that affect the hospital's budget. Although it may be impossible to document the main driver of such staffing changes, nursing and administration often recognize good hospitalist programs as a contributing force.

Physician productivity

Regardless of whether hospitalists are employed by the hospital or by a physician group, the organization will want to see the hospitalists' productivity profile. These profiles often focus on objective encounter and revenue data.

However, hospitalists make contributions to the hospital outside these two areas.

Hospitals often fail to measure and understand the affect hospitalists have on patient flow; fixed and variable costs; quality of care and patient safety; and patient, physician, and nursing satisfaction.

In fact, many hospitals measure hospitalists' contributions to the organization by focusing on physician productivity data. But in regard to such data, hospitalists' overall effectiveness score may be low even when physician productivity is high. Hospital leaders struggle to understand this balance.

Hospitalists should work with nursing and medical staff leaders to ensure accurate assessment of their contributions. As evident from the discussion above, hospitalists should not spend all their time on patient encounters and generating direct revenue. **Figure 2.5** provides a sample "balance sheet" for hospitalist programs. When determining hospitalists' compensation, the discussion should focus on direct patient care, the benefits and outcomes of the program, and overhead costs.

As hospitals and hospitalists begin to consider areas of effectiveness, some data will not yet be available for evaluation. However, it's important for hospitalists and hospital leaders to implement effective measurement systems so, as the hospitalist program matures, the data is captured and analyzed. Remember that although the seven areas of effectiveness discussed above represent positive change, organizations must be prepared to confront some initial frustration and disagreement regarding the accuracy of such data.

How to make the investment

Once the hospital understands how to measure hospitalists' effectiveness, it can examine how to best to invest in a hospitalist program. Although the specifics of contractual arrangements between hospitals and hospitalists will vary for each organization, all hospitals should address several key issues before entering into such relationships.

Remember that hospital and physician relationships often struggle because the two groups fail to discuss important topics before entering into a contract —which creates a strained relationship that revolves around power and control.

Hospitalists should familiarize themselves with the hospital's existing medical staff, nursing staff, and operations, and work with hospital leaders to answer the following questions:

What are the employment options?

Although there are numerous employment models in regard to hospitalists, most fall into the following three categories:

- **Hospitalists directly employed by the hospital**

  Hospitals may employ hospitalists associated with an employed primary care or intensivists practice. In this case, the hospital will ideally negotiate the hospitalists' salary and incentives based on a rational effectiveness plan as described above. In this model, a senior medical officer or operational leader is often held accountable for the hospitalists' performance.

- **Hospitalists employed by an existing private practice**
  In this case, the hospital contracts with a private practice group for defined services but the hospitalists' salary is paid by the practice group.

- **Hospitalists own their own practice group and contract with the hospital**
  Although practical experience has not yet proven this model to be the most effective, it does appropriately base hospitalists' salary and incentives on individual performance.

What key links are needed?

Hospitalists must understand the needs of the key medical practices working at the hospital and create a realistic plan to address those needs. To gain this insight, hospitalists must spend time with the medical staff beyond day-to-day care interaction. In addition, the structure and aim of the hospitalist program must effectively address the quality improvement standards and goals set forth by the medical staff and governing board.

Hospitalists should also establish relationships with the hospital's care management team. The care management team, which includes social workers and care coordinators, are often the first to identify delays and bottlenecks in the delivery of patient care. Hospitalists can be important case management partners by working with medical staff and hospital administration to change processes and redirect resources.

Hospitalists should also establish partnerships with the following departments:

- **Nursing and operations**

  This group usually manages all clinical departments and determines clinical staffing. The activities and priorities of various nursing units, radiology, laboratory, and cardiac testing all determine how well the hospitalist can do his or her job.

- **Medical informatics**

  Many hospitals are developing medical informatics, which provide hospitalists with vital information regarding resource utilization. These systems can also help hospitalists identify improvement opportunities.

- **Medical and patient education**

  Education promotes effective care and provides hospitalists with an opportunity to build their presence and credibility with patients and medical staff members.

Hospitals are complex organizations and accountability is often lost. Hospitalists must strive to establish connections with other practitioners and hospital personnel and assume accountability when appropriate.

At one extreme, hospitalists are simply hired to productively help with hospital care. In such situations, they have weak connections to hospital operations and the medical staff. Although this model allows hospitalists to provide good patient care, their ability to improve hospital operations and medical practices will be limited.

Hospitalists function in a three-dimensional world of patient care, hospital operations, and physician practices. Hospitalists limited to one dimension are unable to effectively improve quality and patient care.

How should salary and incentives be structured?

Regardless of whether hospitalists are employed or contracted, the hospital should tie compensation to the effectiveness measures discussed earlier in this chapter. The medical field continues to debate just how much of a hospitalist's salary should be fixed and how much should be incentive-driven. This determination often depends on the hospitalists' experience and the organization's trust in the effectiveness data.

How much support is needed?

Few hospitalists earn their entire income from their own medical practice. Although physician groups occasionally take on this fiscal responsibility, hospitals are most often responsible to provide some support to the hospitalists.

The hospital, medical staff, and hospitalists must determine the appropriate balance between productivity—based on patient encounters and charges—and developing the hospitalist program and improving relationships with one another. It is clear that hospitalists' time spent on the latter will boost their effectiveness. Turn to **Figure 2.6** for a sample of how a hospital can determine how much support to offer the hospitalist program. This sample clearly takes the bias that support is necessary, and that the value of hospitalists' outcome-related activities must be considered.

It's important for hospitals and hospitalists work together to develop effectiveness measures, carefully examine existing medical and operational policies, and implement a rational salary and incentive structure. The hospital must determine that the hospitalist program will ensure the successful evolution of the acute care process and benefit all key stakeholders. The success of the hospitalist program affects other important hospital initiatives, including wellness, prevention, chronic disease management, and end of life care. Although the use of hospitalists is a fairly new development, these practitioners present numerous opportunities for hospitals, patients, and physicians. Given the centric nature of this work, hospitalists should be well integrated into medical and operational efforts to capture these opportunities.

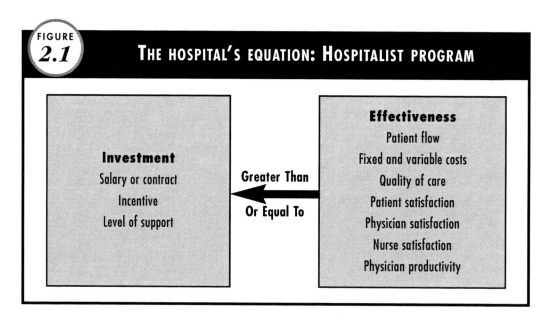

FIGURE
2.1

THE HOSPITAL'S EQUATION: HOSPITALIST PROGRAM

Investment
Salary or contract
Incentive
Level of support

Greater Than
Or Equal To

Effectiveness
Patient flow
Fixed and variable costs
Quality of care
Patient satisfaction
Physician satisfaction
Nurse satisfaction
Physician productivity

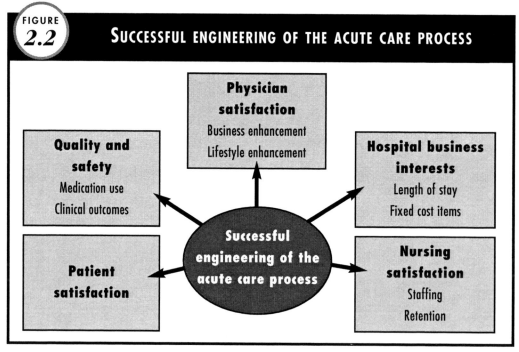

FIGURE
2.2

SUCCESSFUL ENGINEERING OF THE ACUTE CARE PROCESS

Physician satisfaction
Business enhancement
Lifestyle enhancement

Quality and safety
Medication use
Clinical outcomes

Hospital business interests
Length of stay
Fixed cost items

Successful engineering of the acute care process

Patient satisfaction

Nursing satisfaction
Staffing
Retention

FIGURE 2.3 — THE INSTITUTE OF MEDICINE'S 20 QUALITY PRIORITIES

- Care coordination
- Self-management/Health literacy
- Asthma
- Cancer screening
- Children with special care needs
- Diabetes
- End of life with advance system organ failure
- Frailty of old age
- Hypertension
- Immunization
- Ischemic heat disease
- Major depression
- Medication management
- Nosocomial infections
- Pain control in advanced cancer
- Pregnancy and childbirth
- Severe and persistent mental illness
- Stroke
- Tobacco dependence
- Obesity

FIGURE 2.4 — QUALITY PRIORITIES: EXAMPLES FOR HOSPITALIST'S ACTIONS

Medication management
- Insulin administration for diabetes
- Most effective antibiotics for community-acquired and hospital-acquired pneumonia
- Application of effective pain control for a select population or select patient care unit
- Effective anticoagulation initiation and maintenance

Frailty of old age
- Identification and prevention of dementia
- Adequate discharge planning

FIGURE 2.5

HOSPITALIST BALANCE SHEET

Direct patient care
- Average daily census
- Admissions, consultations, and daily encounters
- Net revenue collected

Benefits/outcomes of program
- Quality and efficiency of care markers
- Protocols and standardization developed
- Medical staff and practice group needs met
- Nursing and patient satisfaction
- Electronic medical records development
- Medical education

Program overhead
- Hospitalists' salaries and benefits
- Direct support (nursing, clerical, space)
- Office support (billing, etc.)

FIGURE 2.6

HOSPITAL-BASED HOSPITALISTS PROGRAM: SCENARIO FOR SUPPORT

1. Create a balance sheet for the program. (See Figure 2.5.)

2. Base salary for hospitalists set by examining local and national benchmarks

3. Create incentive for hospitalists
- Must achieve agreed on baseline productivity in patient care work (daily census, encounters, etc.).
- Bonus up to 30% of base salary after evaluation of practice productivity and program benefit. Bias is to favor program outcomes (20%) over additional productivity (10%).

* If the program is practice-based, the hospital will negotiate support for the hospitalists' salary and bonus based on the agreed on balance sheet.

THE PATIENT'S PERSPECTIVE: WHAT CONSTITUTES VALUE AND QUALITY TO HOSPITALIZED PATIENTS?

DIANE CRAIG, MD, FACP

Although most physicians view the hospital as their second home, having walked every hallway at all hours of the day and night, to many patients it is a place filled with painful memories. It is easy for physicians to forget this, fall into their own routine, and have their to-do list running through their minds as they meet yet another new patient in the busy emergency department (ED).

It is difficult for physicians to focus on each patient as an individual amidst the interruptions of beepers and curbside consults. Although physicians spend their careers caring for hospitalized patients, they often fail to look at the hospital from the patient's perspective and measure just how well they are meeting the patient's needs.

Patients have a unique eyewitness perspective on how hospitals work. Their feedback can provide physicians with insight into the inefficiencies of the many systems that collide at the point of contact—: the patient. Learning patients' concerns can also shed light on what constitutes value to patients and what contributes or detracts from their confidence and trust in physicians. Patients' fears have increased because of publicized reports that detail the frequency of medical errors.

In fact, the Institute of Medicine (IOM) acknowledged the importance of patients' perspective in designing an improved health care system in its six aims for improvement discussed in its report *Crossing the Quality Chasm: A New Health System for the 21st Century.*

Hospitalists must understand their patients' experiences and use this knowledge to implement hospital systems that work better for both patients and practitioners. This chapter will outline how hospitalists can benefit from understanding their patients' perspectives, discuss what matters most to patients, and provide steps hospitalists can take to improve patients' hospital experience.

The importance of the patient's perspective

The physician perspective: "The wife was impossible. Mr. Mustard never complained about anything, but his wife was completely unreasonable. She would stalk me in the hallways and ask the same questions over and over again. She resisted taking him home, and when she finally agreed, he had a pulmonary embolism on the way out the door! These things always happen to the most difficult patients."

The patient/family perspective: "The doctors wouldn't tell me what was going on. My husband was getting weaker and weaker, and they just gave up on him. They told me I had to take him home, but I couldn't take care of him alone. I needed more help. Then, when they said he had to go, I came to pick him up and he collapsed and died in my arms on the way out of the hospital. He was all I had."

Physicians don't just treat diseases—they also treat patients. Patients each bring with them their social and emotional history in addition to their physical ailments. Physicians who fail to acknowledge and develop a strategy to treat all the aspects of the patient's life—including the patient's family—will likely become frustrated quickly. This failure may also leave the patient and his or her family angry. In such circumstances, the medical care the patient receives may be jeopardized. Even when the care is appropriate, the risk of the family filing a malpractice suit is significantly increased when the physician fails to establish a positive relationship with the patient.

Malpractice and negligent care suits

Although no studies have yet looked at hospitalists' malpractice experience, most of these practitioners feel their risk of being sued is greater than a primary care physician (PCP) practicing in the outpatient setting. This assumption is based on two factors: the acuity of the illnesses treated and the inherent challenges of caring for patients the hospitalist has never met before.

While these challenges do exist, there are also opportunities for the hospitalist that aren't available to the PCP Seeing the patient for the first time allows an unbiased perspective that may bring clinical problems into sharp focus. Hospital patients are also in a vulnerable state due to their medical condition and may be more willing to extend trust to the physician caring for them. In addition, although a hospitalist may treat a patient for only a few days, he or she actually spends more time with the patient during those few days than the PCP does during an outpatient visit.

What many hospitalists may not know is that the risk of malpractice is linked more closely with communication skills than with medical quality. Studies have shown that malpractice claims and payments are not randomly distributed. A review of nonsurgical physicians in Florida found that 85% of malpractice payments were made on behalf of 3% of the physicians. There was no correlation between these suits and the physicians' training or years of experience. In fact, the only predictor of future claims was the prevalence of past claims.

Keep in mind that most patients affected by negligent medical care never file a malpractice claim. Approximately 1% of hospitalized patients are harmed by significant medical error, and less than 2% of these patients file a claim for compensation. What leads some patients to seek resolution for harm while others let it go? Several studies show that patients who sue often report poor communication with their physician. One study found that communication problems were identified in over 70% of malpractice suits. In a study that interviewed mothers of babies who suffered bad outcomes, those who had been cared for by physicians with frequent malpractice claims reported feeling rushed or ignored, receiving inadequate information or advice, and feeling that the physician spent little time with them during their visit. In yet another study, researchers discovered that in 24% of malpractice claims, a patient's decision to sue was prompted by his or her perception that the physician was not completely honest and the courtroom was the only forum in which he or she could find out what went wrong in their treatment.

Hospitalists have the unique opportunity to discover what is important to patients. In addition to minimizing malpractice risk, this understanding can improve patient compliance, health outcomes, and staff and physician satisfaction.

Patient participation

Except as a core value, hospitalists may not feel a direct incentive to improve patients' long-term health outcomes. It is clear, however, that patients with chronic illnesses who fail to take adequate care of themselves will overuse the health care system—the most costly site of which is hospital care. Patients who feel empowered to take part in their health care have better outcomes, both in terms of symptom control and physiologic measures. In addition, several studies show that the quality of physician communication can affect patient care outcomes. A consistent theme in these studies is the development of a shared decision-making process between the physician and the patient.

Practitioners should offer patients an opportunity to participate in the information-sharing process that goes on during the course of their care. Patient participation allows the necessary personal perspective to meld with the biomedical perspective to design an appropriate treatment plan. Although this exchange may seem more appropriate to an outpatient, nonacute setting, most patients in the hospital are able and eager to participate in decisions regarding their health care. Hospitalists can better reach satisfactory outcomes if they are aware of and accommodate the patients' desire to participate in decisions about their health.

Patient care team

Hospitalists are part of a complex care team that, from the patient's perspective, includes all health care providers who comes into the patient's room wearing a uniform. When members of the care team are satisfied with the role they play and the support they receive, patients are more likely to be satisfied with their care.

Bedside nurses are particularly important in patients' overall assessment of their hospital care. This is not surprising when we consider the amount of time patients spend with nurses as compared to the time patients spend with hospitalists and other physicians during a typical day. Although it takes time to develop relationships with nursing and other support staff on the hospital wards, it is well worth hospitalists' time to do so to improve patients' experiences in the hospital. In Japan, patients with hospital stays in the range of one week or less note that the specific item associated with overall satisfaction with the hospitalization was the skill of their nursing care.

Other studies have shown that when programs were implemented to improve patient satisfaction, staff satisfaction also improved. In addition to improving patient satisfaction, the development of a coherent team to provide complicated care also decreases the risk of errors and bad patient outcomes. All practitioners have cared for patients with the assistance of staff who are unfamiliar with the particular unit in which they are working or the patient's medical condition. It makes everything more complicated and time-consuming. By focusing on the patient, physicians can create a work environment that attracts and retains staff who can provide the kind of care patients expect.

Incentives and referrals

The better the care patients receive, the more likely they are to make referrals to the hospital and hospitalist. Depending on the hospitalist group's economic drivers, soliciting more referrals could be seen as either a positive or negative outcome. Fee-for-service programs have a direct incentive to develop a larger referral base. Salaried hospitalists may have a harder time seeing the benefit of a higher patient census.

Directly or indirectly, the happier patients are with the cared provided at the hospital by a particular physician, the more successful both the physician and hospital will be. This correlation will be more evident when the Hospital Quality Information Initiative is adopted nationwide. The initiative—supported by a number of national hospital associations, the Center for Medicare & Medicaid Services (CMS), Joint Commission on Accreditation of Healthcare Organizations, National Quality Forum, and Agency for Healthcare Research and Quality—focuses on a common set of measures and priorities that assesses clinical care as well as patients' experiences of that care. The clinical measures are underway now and relate to acute myocardial infarction, heart failure, and pneumonia. The patient experience measures are being tested in three states and will be incorporated nationwide in the near future.

Ultimately, Medicare reimbursement will be tied to hospital performance in regard to these measures. The program is based on evidence that patients treated at hospitals with high patient-satisfaction scores experience better outcomes. CMS hopes that better health outcomes will lead to lower health care utilization and lower costs to CMS in the long run. Based on this external incentive, hospital administrators are expected to show an increased interest in patient satisfaction surveys, which offers hospitalists a great opportunity to partner with hospital administrators to create a patient-centered care environment.

Time with patients

Hospitalists and outpatient clinicians are often concerned that providing the information and dialogue that patients want will take too much time. However, the experiences of PCPs show that practitioners who responded to emotional clues from their patients were actually able to complete their visits in the same amount or less time than those who didn't. In a study of PCPs without a history of malpractice claims, the average visit length 3.3 minutes longer than their colleagues with a history of claims. In another study, physicians who worked to elicit all of their patients' concerns were less likely to be caught at the end of the visit by patients' last-minute questions. Allowing patients to tell their stories may save time on the whole. A study of physician interruptions in a primary care setting found that patients were allowed to complete the description of their concerns only 28% of the time. Physicians redirected the patient after a mean of 23 seconds. If allowed to finish, patients only continued for another 6 seconds on average. Late-arising concerns were more than twice as common in interviews where patients were not allowed to finish their story.

The availability of electronic medical records provides an opportunity to gather a majority of the patient's past medical history without actually talking to them, which may increase the efficiency of medical management. However, it also creates a higher patient expectation that everyone in the health care system who should have reviewed his or her medical record has reviewed it. Patients no longer expect physicians to ask what condition prompted the patient's visit. Instead, patients expect the physician to state, "I have reviewed your medical record and see that you recently had bypass surgery and also have diabetes. Can you tell me more about how you've been feeling lately and specifically about the chest pain that brought you in today?"

Reputation and feedback

Patients' perspective also comes into play in regard to reputation. Hospitalists must consider the reputation of their program among patients and, based on their feedback, the satisfaction of the PCPs and other consultants whose patients they manage in the hospital.

Hospitalists' reputation among the physicians in the community is largely formed by patients' feedback. A patient's relationship with a hospitalist is very different than his or her relationship with a PCP. Nonetheless, hospitalists must nurture relationships with patients to reap the benefits associated with improved communication between patients and physicians. Improved communication with patients will not only improve the hospitalists' quality of life by decreasing risk of lawsuits and generating greater revenue for the hospitalists and the hospital, but it will also improve patient outcomes.

The factors that matter most to patients

Until very recently, medical researchers have spent little time investigating how patients perceive their hospital care. In 1989, a review of the literature on patients' evaluations of hospital care found that most of the studies were done in the United Kingdom over a decade before. However, the Picker Institute was founded in 1987 with the goal of creating a patient-centered care environment. The institute undertook the challenge of identifying the issues most important to hospitalized patients and their families. From there, they developed tools to solicit feedback from patients regarding these issues, which could be used by the hospital staff to implement change.

The Picker Institute found the following dimensions of care most important to hospitalized patients.

- Respect for patients' values, preferences, and expressed needs

- Coordination and integration of care

- Information and education

- Physical comfort

- Emotional support and alleviation of fear and anxiety

- Involvement of family and friends

- Transition and continuity of care

- Access to care

They also found that parking, food service, and signage did not appear among the top concerns of patients. These "amenities" are often measured and prioritized by hospital leadership, yet there is little evidence that these factors make a real difference to patients. To some degree, patients expect that hospital parking will be difficult and the food will be mediocre. On the other hand, patients also expect caring physicians and hospital staff, as well as coordinated hospital services. When these expectations are not met, patients are greatly disappointed.

An important feature of the Picker survey process is the measurement of specific behaviors instead of general levels of satisfaction. Asking a patient how satisfied he or she was with his or her discharge instructions may lead to a negative response, but that response will not help the health care team decide how to correct the problem. On the other hand, asking a patient whether anyone explained the purpose of his or her discharge medications or the side effects the patient should watch for provides specific feedback that can improve the discharge process.

Although the dimensions of care listed above are important to patients, hospitalists should focus most on patients' desire that physicians respect their values, preferences, and expressed needs.

The patient's perspective: "They told me I'd die if I didn't have my leg amputated. I told them I'm not going to lose my leg!"

Physicians must understand what lies beneath patients' decisions regarding their health. A decision that appears irrational, manipulative, or uneducated is generally based on a well-developed paradigm in the patient's mind. This paradigm may not include sound scientific evidence, but it is based on the patient's experiences, priorities, and beliefs about health and illness. If the patient's view on health and illness are consistent, the practitioner must consider this information during the course of treatment. Patients are not often quick to share their questions or beliefs about health and illness and may need to be prompted by the physician before revealing these details.

Improve physician-patient communication

There are several models physicians can follow to build effective physician-patient communication. For example, the American Academy for the Physician and Patient offers training programs that elaborate on a model embodied in the acronym PEARLS—partnership, empathy, apology/acknowledgement, respect, legitimization, and support. No matter which program a hospitalist group chooses to improve communication with patients, the basic premise remains the same: Despite all the distractions and interruptions, listen and engage with patients and let them know you care.

One of the most challenging discussions physicians can have with a patient is in regard to a medical error. The medical error may be the result of the hospitalist's mistake or it may have occurred outside of the hospital and led to the patient's admission. Medical errors often involve a system breakdown that caused the patient to miss a medication, receive the wrong drug, suffer a complication from a procedure, or undergo the wrong procedure. Patients are very clear about how they expect physicians to handle such errors: They want physicians to inform them of the error.

Patients want to know what happened, why it happened, and what the physician and hospital are going to do to prevent it from happening again. They also want an apology. Many physicians are reluctant to offer an apology, fearing that it represents an admission of guilt. In most cases, until a thorough root cause analysis is done, the true cause of an error is not apparent and an admission of guilt is not appropriate.

However, acknowledgement of genuine human concern is. A physician should tell the patient that he or she is sorry the error occurred, inform the patient that the cause of the error is not yet known, and that the hospital will conduct an investigation. The physician should also assure the patient that the organization will share the result of the investigation with him or her.

Once hospitalists and other practitioners know what patients want, the real work begins. Health care providers must use this knowledge to improve patient care.

Implement a program that meets patients' needs

Hospitalists are challenged to motivate fellow physicians to prioritize patient satisfaction. Too often physicians focus on patient complaints made by "unreasonable" patients and are too easily frustrated by patients who want more of their physicians' time, who want physicians to come when they call and speak to all of their family members.

Organizational priorities, such as encouraging early discharges, occasionally inconvenience the patient and can also add to the tension between physicians and patients. Beyond personal satisfaction, the physician may not be rewarded for spending more time with patients to improve outcomes and patient satisfaction. However, because most hospital patient satisfaction surveys do not measure a patient's satisfaction with an individual physician, gathering data needed to implement an incentive program for individual physicians is challenging.

Despite these challenges, hospitalists can take the lead in improving hospitalized patients' experiences. As leaders of the hospital health care team, hospitalists are in a unique position to influence the behavior of other hospital staff. Hospitalists should act as patient advocates.

To increase the hospital's focus on patient satisfaction, try the following:

- **Enlist the interest of hospitalists in avoiding malpractice claims**
  Although uncommon, most physicians worry about being sued. The

hospital should share literature that discusses the link between communication skills and the risk of a suit with the medical staff. The hospital risk manager should discuss past malpractice cases against the hospital with physicians to provide evidence that the risk of mistakes and bad outcomes is not a theoretical. Provide an opportunity for physicians to discuss the nonclinical issues that lead to malpractice suits as opposed to the purely clinical aspects of care normally discussed in peer review.

- **Make patient satisfaction an important quality measure**
  As the hospital's primary customer, patients can provide valuable feedback. Ensure that patient feedback is incorporated into the hospital's ongoing monitoring reports and shared at all levels of the organization. Tie manager compensation, employee performance feedback, and physician incentives to the results of the patient feedback.

- **Ask patients about their hospital stays and listen to their response**
  Your hospital probably has a patient satisfaction survey. Review the survey to ensure that the questions provide answers that the hospital can act upon. Look for assessments of specific behaviors rather than levels of satisfaction with phases of care. Advocate for the inclusion of questions specific to physician behaviors.

  Share the results of patient satisfaction survey with physicians. Remember that physicians may attempt to rationalize lapses by pointing to problems with the physical plant, staffing, or the patient population. These obstacles must be acknowledged before physicians accept personal responsibility for poor patient satisfaction.

Because a patient's experience is a combination of all the interactions they have while in the hospital, consider discussing the results in an interdisciplinary group. Some surveys contain verbatim comments from patients, which can be an especially powerful way to get a point across to your physicians and other hospital staff.

- **Invest in education**

  It is possible to improve physicians' communication skills through education and practice. The first step is to share patients' feedback regarding their experiences. For physicians with higher-than-average patient complaints, more intensive training is advisable as a risk management intervention.

- **Consider inviting a patient to speak about his or her experience**

  Patients who file a complaint about their health care experience often do so to ensure other patients experience better care. Many patients, when asked, are willing to share their experience in front of a group of staff to accomplish this goal.

  To be effective, the patient should speak about staff and physicians anonymously to avoid embarrassing anyone, and a neutral party should facilitate the discussion. The facilitator can prepare the patient ahead of time by telling him or her how the session will be structured. The facilitator should also ask whether the patient is comfortable taking questions from the audience.

  The audience must also be prepared. Remind physicians that the patient will deliver their history based on their personal experience, and some details may be inaccurate. However, physicians must understand that the patient is recalling his or her experience as clearly as possible.

Physicians can also invite a colleague who has been a patient at the hospital or who had a family member treated at the hospital to share his or her experiences. Fellow physicians have the added credibility of being on both sides of the care relationship. This vantage point allows them to explain that although they understand why things take so long and communication may lapse, it is unnerving to be on the receiving end of care, and they can help physicians see why.

- **Ensure that patients know who is in charge of their care**

  If patients don't know who is in charge because of the multiple hand-offs that occur during the course of care, they often assume that no one is in charge. Patients meet many new people when they enter the hospital and may need help remembering who is on their care team.

  Encourage practitioners to use business cards and consider posting pictures of the hospitalist team in patient rooms. Encourage physicians to introduce themselves to family members; they may be key decision-makers for the patient. Remind physicians to introduce themselves everyday: "I am Dr. Stuart, and I am in charge of your care while you are here. I met you yesterday, but you weren't feeling very well and I wasn't sure whether you'd remember me. How are you feeling today?"

- **Effectively transfer care at discharge**

  A member of the hospitalist team should call patients after discharge to review discharge instructions, make sure they are stable, and ensure that they have scheduled a post-hospital follow-up appointment. Implement a reliable mechanism to obtain discharge summaries and informal reports to PCPs, and alert the physician of any pending test results.

Make sure patients understand discharge instructions by providing written instructions for them to review when they are more relaxed after discharge.

• **Leverage the PCP**

Hospitalists should recognize the role that the PCP has in determining patient satisfaction with their hospital stay. Work hard to ensure that these practitioners have the information they need to resume post-hospital care.

Hospitalists should make their relationship with patients' PCPs clear. For example, "I work with Dr. Chambers and take care of her patients when they are in the hospital. While she probably won't be able to see you in the hospital, I will make sure she has all the information she needs to care for you. I will also schedule you an appointment with her for follow-up care."

• **Provide resources to help with difficult patients**

Hospitalists and other staff should have ready access to people who can help them when patient interactions go badly. Social workers, discharge planners, psychologists, administrative leaders, risk managers, security officers, and chaplains can all be very helpful in resolving misunderstandings and uncovering the reasons why patients and their families are not happy. Issues of compliance with practitioners' orders and unrealistic expectations may be due to complicated social and emotional challenges that need to be addressed before an appropriate plan of care can be implemented.

PCPs are a very important resource that hospitalists sometimes overlook. Often a simple phone call from the PCP to the patient can reassure the patient and get a plan of care implemented efficiently.

- **Develop an effective approach for disclosing mistakes to patients**
  Every hospitalist must know how to communicate medical errors to patients and share the data patients want to know. The hospitalist group should review the hospital's risk management procedure for handling medical errors to ensure that it meets the group's needs.

- **Select physicians who value patients' perspective**
  Most interview processes do not include an assessment of this dimension of a physician's accomplishments. However, an assessment of the candidate's overall demeanor may indicate a commitment to patient satisfaction. Keep in mind that all physicians are on their best behavior during an interview and may take one approach to dealing with other professionals and another for dealing with patients. Consider including support staff in your interview process; how candidates interact with support staff may shed light on how they will interact with patients.

Hospitalists may also build a patient satisfaction question into the interview. Ask the candidate to remember a difficult patient interaction and how they handled it. Look for evidence that the physician took responsibility for how they contributed to the problem, went the extra mile for the patient, and looked for innovative solutions.

• **Build patient satisfaction into performance evaluations**
To ensure that hospitalists and other practitioners prioritize patient satisfaction, it must be effectively measured and incorporated into compensation evaluations. In addition, less formal means of recognizing good patient care are also important, including celebratory lunches and parties to reward staff and physicians for their hard work in caring for patients.

• **Adopt a culture that puts the patient first**
Improving patient satisfaction does not require facility renovations, extra staff, or elaborate computer networks. Hospitals' only investment is in their practitioners. Hospital leaders, including the leaders of the hospitalist program, must remind practitioners that patients are the organization's top priority. Patients will notice when a hospital incorporates their preferences into the design of its systems.

References

Barnett, P.B., "Rapport and the hospitalist," *American Journal of Medicine* 2001; 111(9B): 31S–35S.Gerteis, M., S. Edgman-Levitan, et al., *Through the Patient's Eyes: Understanding and Promoting Patient-Centered Care.* San Francisco. Jossey-Bass, 1993.

Barrier, P.A., J.T. Li, and N.M. Jensen, "Two words to improve physician-patient communication: What else?" *Mayo Clin Proc.* February 2003; 78(2):211–214. Beckman, H.B. et al., "The doctor-patient relationship and malpractice: Lessons from plaintiff depositions," *Arch Intern Med.* 1994;154:1365–1370.

Brennan, T.A., L.L. Leape, N.M. Laird, "Incidence of adverse events and negligence in hospitalized patients: Results of Harvard Medical Practice Study I," *New England Journal of Medicine.* 1991; 324:370-376.

Cleary, P.D., S. Edgman-Levitan, et al., "Patients Evaluate Their Hospital Care: A National Survey," *Health Aff.* 1991;10(4):254–67.

Delbanco, T., "Hospital Medicine: Understanding and Drawing on the Patient's Perspective," *American Journal of Medicine.* 2001;111(9B): 2S–4S.

Entman, S.S., C.A. Glass, et al.. "The relationship between malpractice claims history and subsequent obstetric care," *Journal of the American Medical Association.* 1994;272: 1588–1591.

Fremont, A.M., P.D. Cleary, et al., "Patient-centered Processes of Care and Long-Term Outcomes of Myocardial Infarction," *J Gen Intern Med.* 2001;16:800-808.

Gallagher, T.H., A.D. Waterman, et al., "Patients' and Physicians' Attitudes Regarding the Disclosure of Medical Errors," *Journal of the American Medical Association.* 2003;289:1001–1007.

Greenfield, S., S.H. Kaplan, J.E. Ware, et al., "Patients' participation in medical care: Effects on blood sugar control and quality of life in diabetes," *J Gen Intern Med.* 1988;3:448–457.

Haidet D. and D.A. Paterniti, " 'Building ' a History Rather Than 'Taking' One. A perspective on information sharing during the medical interview,". *Arch Intern Med* 2003;163:1134-1140.

Hickson, G.B., C.F. Federspiel, et al, "Patient complaints and malpractice risk," *Journal of the American Medical Association.* June 12, 2002. 12;287(22):2951–7.

Hickson, G.B., E.W. Clayton, et al., "Factors that prompted families to file medical malpractice claims following perinatal injuries," *Journal of the American Medical Association.* 1992;267:1359–1363.

Hickson, G.B., E.W. Clayton, et al., "Obstetricians' prior malpractice experience and patients' satisfaction with care," *Journal of the American Medical Association.* 1994;272:1583–1587.

IOM's Committee on Quality of Health Care in America. *Crossing the Quality Chasm: A New Health System for the 21st Century.* Washington, DC: National Academy Press, 2001.

IOM's Committee on Quality of Health Care in America. *To Err is Human: Building a Safer Health System.* Washington, DC: National Academy Press, 2000.

Kaplan, S.H., S. Greenfield, and J.E. Ware, "Assessing the effects of physician-patient interactions on the outcomes of chronic disease," *Med Care.* 1989;27:S110–S127.

Kielhorn, T.M., "Reducing Risk by Improving Communication," *The Permanente Journal.* 1997;1(1): 69–70.

Levinson, W., D.L. Roter, et al., "Physician-patient communication: The relationship with malpractice claims among primary care physicians and surgeons," *Journal of the American Medical Association.* February 19, 1997;277(7):553–9.

Levinson, W., R. Goraware-Bhat, and J. Lamb, "A study of patient clues and physician responses in primary care and surgical settings," *Journal of the American Medical Association.* August 23–30, 2000;284(8):1002–7.

Localio, A.R., A.G. Lawthers, T.A. Brennan, et al., "Relationship between malpractice claims and adverse events due to negligence: Results of the

Harvard Medical Practice Study III," *New England Journal of Medicine.* 1991;325:245–251.

Marvel, M.K., R.M. Epstein, et al., "Soliciting the patient's agenda: Have we improved?" *Journal of the American Medical Association.* January 20, 1999;281(3):283–7

May, M.L. and D.B. Stengel, "Who sues their doctors? How patients handle medical grievances," *Law Society Review.* 1990;24(1):105–120.

Roter, D.L. and J. Hall, "Improving physicians' interviewing skills and reducing patients' emotional distress: A randomized clinical trial," *Arch Intern Med.* 1995;155:1877–1884.

Rubin, H.R., "Patient evaluations of hospital care. A review of the literature," *Med Care.* 1989;28(9 Suppl):S3–9.

Sloan, F., E.M. Mergenhagen, et al., "Medical malpractice experience of physicians: Predictable or haphazard?" *Journal of the American Medical Association.* 1989;262:3291–3297

Stewart, M.A., "Effective physician-patient communication and health outcomes: A review," *CMAJ.* 1995;152:1423-1433.

Tokunaga J. and Y. Imanaka, "Influence of length of stay on patient satisfaction with hospital care in Japan," *Int J Qual Health Care.* 2002 Dec;14(6):493–502

Witman, A.B., D.M. Park, and S.B. Hardin. "How do patients want physicians to handle mistakes," *Arch Intern Med.* 1996;156:2565–69.

White, J., W. Levinson, and D. Roter, "Oh, by the way…". *J Gen Intern Med.* 1994;9:24–28.

Systems of Operation 1: Communication—The key to a sound hospitalist program

Leslie E. Cowan, RN, BSN

Jeffrey R. Dichter, MD, FACP

Editor's note: Behind every good hospitalist program is a sound system for its implementation and operation. Chapters 4 and 5 focus on how to build a strong program. Specifically, this chapter covers communication, while Chapter 5 covers coordination of care, data evaluation, and customer satisfaction.

Identify your 'customers'

Communication is the single most important component of a successful hospitalist program. The increasing number of hospitalists in the United States demands greater attention to the communication processes between hospitalists and primary care physicians (PCP), and hospitalists and patients. Levels of communication vary based on the needs of each group of customers. The three most important groups of customers with which hospitalists interact are primary care and referring physicians, nursing and other inpatient professionals, and patients and families.

Determine who your customers are and form appropriate means of communicating with them. Define their needs and expectations, and then build the system around them. Find out what your customers want by formally surveying them, as well as by engaging them in simple discussions.

Develop and adhere to a predefined set of procedures and protocols for each customer group. Put these procedures, protocols, and expectations in writing and provide them to all customers and stakeholders.

Establish communication mechanisms

Mechanisms for requesting hospitalist services

Discussion between hospitalists and other physicians is arguably the most important communication link in a hospitalist program. Therefore, hospital policy should clearly define how other physicians, physician office staffs, or emergency department (ED) physicians might access this service.

When building a system, first gather feedback from these physicians. Some of the most commonly employed mechanisms through which other physicians contact hospitalists include the following:

- The referring physician or office staff pages the hospitalist to inform him or her of the requested admission or consultation. The advantage of this mechanism is that the hospitalist has an opportunity to speak directly with the referring physician or staff member. The disadvantage is that it requires the referring office staff to depend on a return call from the hospitalist, thereby risking delayed or missed notification.

- The referring physicians or office staff call in their request to the hospitalist's office or an admissions coordinator or his or her administrative equivalent. This individual is responsible for notifying the hospitalist of the patient that he or she must see. This mechanism makes it easy and quick for referring physicians to request hospitalist assistance. The downside is there may be no direct communication between the referring physician or office staff and the hospitalist.

- The ED directly notifies the on-call hospitalist via pager or telephone.

- Urgent or emergency requests require direct communication between the referring physician or designee and hospitalist. This mechanism is analogous to how an ED would access a hospitalist.

Regardless of which mechanisms are used, it is crucial that they are communicated to referring physicians, their office staff, ED(s), page operators, and all other key personnel. Communication procedures must be reinforced over time, given the typical turnover of personnel in health care venues.

Mechanisms for communicating with referring physicians

If a hospitalist needs patient information from a referring physician's office, there should be a mechanism for requesting this information. Such a mechanism might include a formal method for requesting documents (e.g., have administrative personnel call) and a checklist of the types of information needed. Typical office information requests include a recent medical history and physical exam, a current list of medications and allergies, and recent lab tests or x-ray reports.

Don't forget to spell out the accepted methods for delivering office information (e.g., fax, e-mail, snail mail, etc.).

Communication during patient hospitalization

What information PCPs want to see during a patient's hospitalization will vary. Knowing their preferences is important to construct this part of a program's communication, as discussed above.

Key information most PCPs will want to know is whether significant or unexpected clinical deterioration occurs, any change in code status, or if conflict arises between caregivers and patients or family. These types of circumstances might warrant the PCP's involvement.

Post-discharge communication

In arriving at a procedure for post-discharge communication, it is again important to know what your PCPs want. Some of the commonly identified discharge information needs include the following:

- PCPs need to know when their patients are being discharged, as well as what happened during the hospitalization. A telephone call from the hospitalist is a common way to impart this information.

- PCPs usually prefer to receive a formal discharge summary. Most hospitals have discharge summaries dictated and faxed or mailed to the primary-care physician's office. Ideally, this information should be turned around in short order so the PCP receives it the same day as the discharge. If this timing is not possible, the hospitalist service could prepare a brief, even handwritten discharge summary that could be faxed, e-mailed, or otherwise sent to a PCP's office that day. Any discharge summary should include a list of a patient's diagnoses, medications, key diagnostic tests, and any other data the PCP desires.

- In addition to the required elements, other key items addressed at discharge include new diagnoses and supporting criteria or data; other diagnostic tests performed; changes in medication regimens; changes in diet and rationale; and carefully outlined discharge plans and follow-up, especially tests such as x-rays, blood tests, etc.

- If discharge summaries are sent via fax from the hospital, verify that all referring physicians have fax machines, and if/when they turn them off. It may be worthwhile to keep a log of where and when each discharge is faxed or otherwise sent, to help verify its receipt.

- Patients often have difficulty with discharge instructions and plans. Informing the primary-care physician verbally and noting in the discharge summary any key follow-up issues help optimize patient follow-up and compliance.

- It's helpful for hospitalists to make a single, daily telephone call to PCPs for updates and discharges. But due to the nature of hospital work, this may not always be possible.

- Provide each patient with a copy of his or her own discharge summary, as he or she is apt to bring it along to follow-up appointments.

Communication with patients during hospitalization

Diane Craig has done an excellent job of describing patient needs during hospitalization (see **Chapter 3**). But hospitalists need to focus on a few additional information needs to increase patient and family satisfaction.

Many patients and families have never been exposed to hospitalists before, and therefore may not understand how these professionals function. Establishing appropriate and realistic expectations from the outset is imperative. To that end, organizations may require that all hospitalists give a brief, standard description of the hospitalist service upon introducing themselves to a patient. This description should be defined by each group of hospitalists and standardized so patients and families receive the same information.

Most patients also appreciate regular feedback regarding their progress. It is important that hospitalists explain to patients what is planned for them, and what they might expect. It is particularly important to inform them of when they can expect to be discharged.

In addition to setting realistic expectations, hospitalists should have a standard process that allows patients and families reach them. This process might include meeting at the bedside at an agreed-upon time, having the nursing staff page the hospitalist when family is available, or another defined mechanism.

Although hospitalists will often see patients two or more times per day, a service may elect to provide a standard daily follow-up visit for all patients. These visits may allow opportunities to discuss tests conducted earlier in the day. Although two daily visits may be inconvenient for a busy service, it is a powerful mechanism for gaining the confidence and support of patients and family.

A hospitalist service brochure is another powerful way to communicate with patients and families. A well-designed brochure will answer many of their questions, possibly forestalling anxiety and misunderstandings. Some of the information included in a brochure may include the following:

- How the program functions

- How to contact hospitalists

- The benefits of the program

- How it is designed to meet the needs of patients and families

- Expectations the service may have of patients during their hospitalization

- How hospitalists interact with PCPs

- Expectations for patients after discharge (e.g., when to follow-up with their PCP)

- A picture and brief biography of each hospitalist—including education, training, and credentials information, as these are items of increasing importance to the public)

Communication with patients at discharge and beyond

The discharge process should be clearly defined for patients. Most hospitals have a defined process that usually includes discharge documents, counseling, and perhaps sending home some medications (e.g., multidose inhalers). Having a complete discharge process is particularly important for hospitalist services in optimizing patient follow-up with PCPs and other physicians. Hospitalist services should have follow-up plans clearly documented and understood by patients and physician offices whenever possible.

Although many hospitalists have little contact with patients after discharge, there are two post-discharge opportunities worth discussing. In some environments, it may be worthwhile to make space available for occasional follow-up appointments. The purpose of such appointments may be, for instance, to check blood pressure or a wound. The purpose(s) of a follow-up visit should be clearly defined in advance and may include necessary follow-up to facilitate an early discharge, or provide routine care until a patient can receive the necessary long-term follow-up. Hospitalist practices may offer this service in an office environment, if available; some programs use ED space.

A two- to three-day post-discharge telephone call from the hospitalist to the patient is also an appropriate standard. The call would verify whether a patient is functioning well at home, received his or her medicines or medical equipment, and scheduled necessary follow-up appointments. Post-discharge follow-up is a powerful tool to enhance patient compliance. It is also an effective marketing tool, as patients greatly appreciate when their doctors call them. Follow-up calls may be placed by a case manager or other staff member, but carry more weight when done by a physician. Providing hospitalists with a copy of the discharge summary and a telephone number facilitates call completion.

Contact with outside organizations

Outside organizations are likely to contact hospitalist practices after patient discharge. Such organizations include pharmacies with questions regarding scripts or other discharge supplies, home care agencies looking for clarifications or signed orders, mortuaries looking for the appropriate physician to sign death certificates, etc. Although most inquiries may be deferred elsewhere, hospitalist practices should have a mechanism for responding promptly.

Communication with nursing and other inpatient professionals

Communication with other inpatient professionals is a crucial part of hospitalist service. Although nursing is particularly important, connecting with other professionals (e.g., pharmacy, physical/occupational/speech therapy, dietary, radiology, etc.) is just as crucial. Poor working relationships among interdisciplinary team members could have a negative effect on patient care and the teaching environment.

The following are strategies for effective communication and collaboration:

- Respectfulness

- Professionalism

- Active listening

- Understanding others' viewpoints

- Acknowledgement of others' thoughts and feelings

- Cooperation

- Looking for shared concerns

- Stating one's own opinions and feelings

- Acknowledging when one is wrong

- Postulating possible solutions before meetings

- Viewing conflict resolution as a helical process.

One strategy for improving group communication is to hold a daily team meeting. Such meetings bring everyone together to discuss patient issues and give multidisciplinary input. But a disadvantage to daily meetings is that they require a great deal of coordination and team members' time and resources.

If a team meeting is not possible, there should be some mechanism for regular interaction with the other inpatient professionals. Whatever mechanism you choose, it should become a part of your hospitalist service's formal expectations and standards.

Monitor communication

In an ideal world, all health care organizations would systematically monitor all forms of communication to stay abreast of how effectively a service performs. However, such an endeavor is difficult and time/resource-consuming. There are many moving parts, the means to measure them are not always well defined, and finding meaningful feedback loops can be difficult. However, there are some ways a hospitalist program can obtain feedback about the effectiveness of its communication.

Send physicians a periodic (perhaps annual) survey on which they have a chance to evaluate hospitalist performance. See **Figure 4.1** for a sample survey. Physician feedback can also be gathered in less formal ways, such as via a periodic phone call. Also survey nurses and other professionals this way.

Obtaining feedback from patients is more difficult, however. Although most hospitals have sophisticated means to measure patient satisfaction after discharge, rarely does it provide meaningful feedback on hospitalists. Hospitalists should check with their institutions to see what data are available. Exit/ discharge interviews with a sampling of patients may be another mechanism to gain information.

Tools of communication

A physician's traditional toolbox of communication devices has long been the pager and the telephone, and perhaps a fax machine. Hospitalists, by their relative youth and the nature of their work, are technologically savvy. The availability of technological tools is now much greater and growing rapidly. Some of these new tools include the following:

- Cellular telephones

- Alpha-numeric pagers with sophisticated digital reception

- Personal digital assistants, often with wireless two-way communication

- Web-based applications to access patient information

- Telemedicine

It is important for each service to determine which tools will work best for it in the present environment and in the near future. The capabilities and expectations of their own practices and hospitals and those of referring physicians and patients will govern technology choices. Emerging technologies promise to offer hospitalist practices powerful new tools to improve the quality and efficiency of their work.

Resources

Farley, Tony and Steve Slutzky. "The Electronic Option: Case Report," *Healthcare Informatics*, July 2003. Online resource: *www. healthcare-informatics.com.*

Middleton, Greg R.., "Tapping the Potential of Paging," *EMS:* 81–84, 90; August 2002.

Nelson, John R., "The Importance of Post Discharge Telephone Follow-up for Hospitalists: A View from the Trenches," *The American Journal of Medicine*, Volume 111: 43S–44S; December 2001

Nelson, John R. and Winthrop F. Whitcomb, "Organizing a hospitalist program: an overview of fundamental concepts," *Medical Clinics of North America*, 86: 4; 887–909; July 2002.

Rider, Elizabeth, "Twelve strategies for effective communication and collaboration in medical teams," *British Medical Journal*, 325: S45; August 2002.

FIGURE 4.1

HOSPITALIST SURVEY: MEDICAL CONSULTANTS

Practice _____

Name (optional) _____

	Strongly agree				Strongly disagree

1. I find the hospitalist service valuable. 1 2 3 4 5

Comments

_____
_____

2. When consulted, the hospitalist physicians are easily available. 1 2 3 4 5

Comments

_____
_____

3. When consulted, the hospitalist physician's are professional and courteous. 1 2 3 4 5

Comments

_____
_____

FIGURE 4.1 — **HOSPITALIST SURVEY: MEDICAL CONSULTANTS (CONT.)**

	Strongly agree				Strongly disagree

4. I feel my patients have been well cared for as
   hospitalist patients.   1 2 3 4 5

Comments

_____

_____

5. My patients were satisfied with the care provided by
   the hospitalist physician.   1 2 3 4 5

Comments

_____

_____

6. Upon discharge, I received a telephone call with a
   thorough update on patient's discharge condition and plan.   1 2 3 4 5

Comments

_____

_____

FIGURE 4.1   **HOSPITALIST SURVEY: MEDICAL CONSULTANTS (CONT.)**

	Strongly agree				Strongly disagree

7. The discharge summary I received via fax provides a complete picture of the hospital stay and discharge plan.   1   2   3   4   5

Comments

_____

_____

8. What could be improved about the hospitalist service that would better meet your needs?   1   2   3   4   5

Comments

_____

_____

9. General comments:

_____

_____

_____

_____

_____

_____

_____

_____

Systems of Operation 2: Coordination of care, data evaluation, and customer satisfaction

Leslie E. Cowan, RN, BSN

Jeffrey R. Dichter, MD, FACP

A modern hospitalist program requires interdependence and teamwork, as well as a defined, solid administrative structure to support key functions such as coordination of care, data evaluation, customer satisfaction, and marketing.

Overview of program needs: Support personnel

Most hospitalist practices are busy and quickly growing. Physician time is best spent seeing patients and recruiting new hospitalists. Therefore, hospitalist practices should employ support personnel to manage the key functions listed above.

Most programs assign a medical director to be responsible for oversight of these functions. He or she is often paid a stipend, and some hospitalist groups provide the medical director with substantial time during normal work hours to carry out these responsibilities. Therefore, it is important for hospitalist groups to clearly define key functions and identify support personnel.

Each program must decide for itself the level of support personnel it requires. Small practices may have only a nurse, case manager, or designated administrator to perform these duties. However, a large practice or hospitalist company may have teams of designated personnel for each function.

To determine the level of support required, a hospitalist program must identify the key areas of need, and define responsibilities and accountabilities. Keep in mind that support personnel should be familiar with the hospitalist practice, its key customers, and the hospital(s) it serves.

Support personnel ideally should work in an office located either in or near the primary hospital served.

Though the equipment needed for an office may seem obvious, it should include a fax machine, a computer system connected to the hospital's information system, telephones, cell phones, pagers, desks, mail boxes, and a filing system. An answering service, clerical support, and some form of office support are also needed if the program has a preoperative clinic or provides post-discharge care.

Coordination of care

Hospitalist practices typically require more interdependence and coordination than other physician practices. The inpatient workload is unpredictable at best and caring for inpatients is more labor-intensive than providing consultation services. Hospitalist practices must implement systems to manage these heavy workloads.

Hospitalist to hospitalist

A busy hospitalist service may admit and provide consultative services to as many as 25 new patients a day. Only one or two hospitalists cannot care for so many new patients while treating established patients. In addition, the unpredictable ebb and flow of patients may result in significant disparities regarding the number of patients each hospitalist is assigned.

Most hospitalist experts believe that a daily patient census of more than 20 may result in declined efficiency and quality. However, this challenge is difficult to overcome. The traditional physician culture poses one of the toughest obstacles in regard to patient census. For example, physicians often equate being on call with the responsibility to treat all new patients—asking physicians who are not on call for help may be interpreted as weakness. Therefore, hospitalist services should have defined mechanisms for optimizing and sharing workloads.

The goal of optimizing workloads is to equalize hospitalist censuses as much as possible, either by distributing admissions and consultations to all hospitalist team members, or redistributing workloads by implementing other means such as the following:

1. **Routinely sharing admissions across the group.** It is helpful to have an established expectation, for instance

   • the hospitalist who is not on call may be expected to take a specified number (perhaps two or three) of new patients (admissions or consults) daily.

   • the on-call hospitalist should assign new patients since he or she is typically the practitioner contacted for new patients. This function could also be performed by a nurse, case manager, or other responsible professional.

2. **Implementing a mechanism for distributing work when the volume of patients between hospitalists differs significantly.** However, this poses its own challenges because the admitting hospitalist, who may know the patient best, will not provide ongoing care. Therefore

   • to optimize continuity of care, reassignment of patients should occur as early in the admission as possible

   • reassignment of patients should occur as few times as possible, whether for team workload needs, vacation, etc.

Note: Reassignment of new admissions or consultations routinely occurs in programs that utilize a night float system (see **Chapter 6** for more information). It also occurs in virtually every practice when a physician goes on vacation, or is otherwise unavailable.

3. **Establishing a goal for the maximum number of patients that each hospitalist should care for at one time** (typically 20–30). Although it is not always possible to comply with this goal, establishing a limit helps hospitalists focus on maintaining an appropriate patient census.

4. **Establishing a mechanism for signing over patients to on-call hospitalists, whether for an evening or an extended period of time**

5. **Determining a standard timeframe in which new admissions or consultations are seen.** Again, it is unrealistic to expect that any service will achieve perfect compliance with such a standard, but it does keep the team focused on it as a goal.

Hospitalists with other professionals

To optimize efficiency and maintain quality, hospitalists often require a means to facilitate patients' care throughout the day—despite the inevitability of not seeing many of their patients until late in the day.

Though much of this communication between caregivers occurs by happenstance (the conversations in the hallway), it is more effective to have a systematic mechanism in place. For example, holding a daily team meeting or assigning case managers to function as intermediaries between hospitalists and other disciplines.

A daily meeting may be a brief get-together for physicians, or it may be a formal meeting that involves many other inpatient disciplines. In addition to the workload issues addressed above, a daily meeting allows physicians a chance to discuss difficult patient care issues and receive updates about administrative issues. A multidisciplinary team meeting allows professionals to share their perspectives on key or difficult issues. Remember, hospitalists often interact with nursing, pharmacy, respiratory/physical/occupational/ speech therapy, and case management personnel. Hospitalists should have a clearly defined expectation of what information is required from each discipline.

Keep in mind that the goal of daily meetings is to implement a system to effectively communicate patient care decisions and information to appropriate patient care wards or caregivers.

Case managers assigned to hospitalists can also facilitate communication and care among hospitalists and other inpatient professionals. Although case managers have many functions, their key roles include assessing ongoing patient care needs, facilitating efficient coordination of care, and discharge planning.

Assessment of hospitalist program data

The collection and reporting of data is the backbone of any hospitalist group, as it provides a foundation for the assessment of quality and efficiency. The hospitalist group should collect data that allow it to evaluate the performance of the entire program, as well as the performance of individuals.

The data should be regularly reviewed—monthly or quarterly—by the entire group, to give hospitalists an opportunity to learn from each other, look for ways to improve the program, and explore future data needs. Analyzing the data as a group also provides for healthy competition. However, the data should never be used in a punitive manner.

Customer satisfaction

Hospitalists must assess customer satisfaction. As defined in **Chapter 4,** hospitalist program customers include patients, referring physicians, hospitals, nurses, and members of the multidisciplinary team. Assessing the satisfaction of all these customers can be overwhelming.

Patients
Most hospitals have a patient-satisfaction tool that surveys patients or families soon after discharge. However, these routine methods do not always measure satisfaction with the care provided by hospitalists. Hospitalists should work with the hospital to incorporate this aspect of care into the overall patient satisfaction survey. For example, the Society of Hospital Medicine (formerly

the National Association of Inpatient Physicians) at presstime was working with the largest hospital-patient satisfaction survey company to develop a standard "hospital medicine" template.

Referring physicians

Few hospitalist programs have implemented a system to measure referring physician satisfaction. However, we recommend developing a simple survey form that is to mailed referring physicians annually. (Turn to **Chapter 4** for a sample survey.) The questions should be simple and request assessment of satisfaction based on a numeric scale.

Inpatient professionals

Nursing and other multidisciplinary staff who work with the hospitalist program are the final customers to survey in regard to patient satisfaction. Because of the acute shortages in many areas of the hospital work force, hospitalists can play a key role in retaining these team members.

It is also important to keep in mind that this group of professionals can be a powerful marketing force for or against a hospitalist program. Therefore, a short survey, similar to that described above for referring physicians, that is completed on a recurring, scheduled basis, can provide valuable information.

RESOURCE SECURITY: SECURE HOSPITALIST RESOURCES IN A DYNAMIC MARKETPLACE

STACEY GOLDSHOLL, MD

The hospitalist marketplace is one of dynamic fluidity. In 1999, the *American Journal of Medicine* published projections that anticipated a hospitalist work force of over 20,000 by 2010. This projection is twice the number of hospitalists currently practice in the United States. However, some experts expect these projections will be exceeded.

The law of supply and demand places hospitalists in the unique position to design their own career paths. Those who are part of a stable hospitalists program are often lured to other hospitals to establish new programs. Hospitalists are also often in the position to choose more attractive work schedules—opting out of call-based staffing for shift-based models. A market with such high demand motivates these practitioners to seek out ideal career opportunities. The laws of the marketplace, combined with the intense nature of hospitalists' work, makes resource security an essential component of all successful hospitalists programs.

Resource security is difficult to define because it is shaped differently by each organization. The factors that make hospitalists feel secure in their position, ward off attrition, and promote professional satisfaction are affected by the unique characteristics of each hospital. However, in such a fluid work force, hospitals and hospitalist groups cannot overlook the economics of physician recruitment and the disruption of physician turnover.

These organizations must determine what factors secure hospitalists' loyalty and what factors destabilize resource security. The answers to these questions are as individualized as hospitalists themselves. However, this chapter will discuss the common themes that surface when hospitals and hospitalist groups attempt to devise a strategy for resource security.

Patient volume and hospitalist staffing

Hospitalists frequently cite understaffing as a primary reason why they leave one hospitalists program to join another. These physicians are frustrated by the hospitalists group's inability to cover the call schedule, which results in excessive workloads. However, hospitalist groups struggle to define appropriate staffing. To make this determination, the group must consider the staffing model and the volume of patients they must treat.

Patient volume

Poor case-management recordkeeping, disjointed data systems, and unpredictable medical staff utilization of hospitalists make it difficult to anticipate patient volume. However, the importance of volume projection cannot be overstated. Underestimating patient volume can lead to the scenario of too much, too soon. In such situations, newly incorporated hospitalist resources are stressed beyond their limit by an over-abundance of patient care demands, which can quickly lead to the program's failure.

Therefore, an accurate projection of patient volume that includes unassigned emergency department (ED) admissions, annual admission data of private physician enrollment, and medical consultations should be determined in advance of physician recruitment.

The following resources can help uncover admission data:

- **Vice president of medical affairs (VPMA)**
  The VPMA traditionally receives admission data for all medical staff members. The hospitalists program should identify the primary care physicians (PCPs) who will use the hospitalists' services and solicit the VPMA's help gathering data regarding the physicians' admission rates.

- **ED medical director**
  It is often difficult to gather information regarding the frequency of unassigned ED medical admissions. However, hospitalists should partner with the hospital's ED medical director to best estimate the number of such admissions.

- **Critical care nurse manager**

  If the hospitalist group is considering providing 24-hour in-house services, it should contact the critical care nurse manager for information regarding the volume of code blue patient encounters.

- **Clinical resource director**

  Hospitalists should contact the hospital's clinical resource director if the organization has implemented case-management data systems. The clinical resource director may be able to provide information related to inpatient volumes for individual physicians as well as volumes based on diagnosis.

Once the hospitalist group determines the average volume of patient admissions, it should consult national benchmarks regarding average hospitalist workloads to project staffing needs. Interpret this data carefully, however. The definition of a reasonable workload—patient load per physician, hours worked per week, adequate time off, etc.—can be subjective and should be considered in the context of individual program goals and support systems. The Society of Hospital Medicine's 2002 benchmarks task force revealed that in one year the average hospitalist admits a mean of 575 new patient, sees 2300 patients, and works 2100 hours in the hospital. These hours do not include on-call availability. Unfortunately, this data does not indicate the staffing model used by the hospitalists surveyed and does not include data that reflects physician retention and workload sustainability.

However, hospitalists can estimate its need for full-time employees (FTE) based on 600–800 admissions per FTE physician. Keep in mind that the group's staffing model will determine the number of physicians it needs to provide 24 hour in-house or on-call coverage. Therefore, hospitalists should project daily FTE requirements based on average daily census calculations (see formula below).

Keep in mind that external factors will affect hospitalists' workload. Many of these factors are not in physicians' control due to complicated hospital inter-dependent systems and the patient population. These factors include patient acuity, hospitalists' years of experience, the provision of support staff (e.g., office support staff, designated case managers, physician assistants, nurse practitioners), system inefficiencies (e.g., delays in transcription and reporting and entry of physician orders), and hospital bed geography (e.g., more than one hospital to serve or patients scattered throughout a large institution). A hospitalist who partners with a case manager or nurse practitioner may comfortably see 26 patients in a day, while a hospitalist who works alone may have trouble seeing more than 16 patients. All of these factors affect efficiency, productivity, and workload.

Once the number of new admissions and consultations is projected, an average daily census (ADC) can be calculated using the following formula:

$$\frac{\text{Annual admissions/consults x Average length of stay}}{365} = \text{ADC}$$

The ADC can then be used to determine the number of hospitalists needed. For all of the reasons outlined above, determining the appropriate patient-to-physician ratio can be quite a challenge. There is no one number that fits the needs of all programs.

However, hospitalist programs can start this process by looking at a 12-hour day with 12 to 14 patients and two to three new admissions and consultations. This workload is conducive to providing high quality of care while maintaining physician satisfaction. Hospitalists with this workload have the opportunity to develop good communication with PCPs and consulting physicians and visit patients more than once during their shift.

Remember: The ADC should not be used as the sole tool for determining physician workload. Hospitalist groups must also consider that as the length of stay is decreased, physician work increases even though the daily census will decrease. Therefore, individual program goals must be factored into the equation to determine the ideal ratio of patient-load to physician. A good rule of thumb for determining appropriate staffing is dividing the ADC by 15 patients and physicians. Consider the following example:

1. Projected annual admissions = 3200

2. Average length of stay = 5 .1 days

3. ADC

   (3200 annual admissions x 5.1 days/admissions)/365 = 45 patients/day

4. Number of rounding hospitalists = ADC/Workload per physician

   ADC/15 patients per rounding hospitalist = 3 hospitalists/day

After the number of hospitalists needed to attend to patients each day is determined, the number of hospitalists needed for program implementation can be determined based on the staffing model the group chooses.

Staffing models

There are a number of hospitalist staffing models—shifts v. on-call, and weekends/nights v. Monday through Friday. Every hospitalist program requires 24-hour availability, but it must decide to provide that availability by in-house physicians or by physicians on-call. The program's financial and quality goals, and the owner of the hospitalists program will determine which model best suits the organization.

Traditional staffing model

The economic benefits of the traditional staffing model ensures its continued popularity. Hospitalists in this model conduct rounds during the day and are scheduled for on-call duty. It is impossible to predict how often the hospitalist on-call will be required to return to the hospital in the evening, and physicians rotate night availability based on the number of physicians in the call group. In many new hospitalist programs, physicians are required to take on-call duty as frequently as every fourth or fifth night with rotating weekends.

This model is most common in private hospitalist groups, hospitalist management companies, and multispecialty groups. However, the cost of this availability is generally not recognized. Allowing hospitalists to have weekends off creates the need for part-time weekend help or back-up coverage because the patient census will require the same number of rounding physicians. In determining the staffing requirements for the patient census above, consider the following:

ADC = 45

Ideal patient/physician load = 15

Daytime rounding physicians (45 ADC/15 patients) = 3

Daily hours of in-house physician time (3 physicians x 12 hr shift) = 36

Hours/year of physician time (36 hours x 365) = 13,140

Hours/FTE (2100 + 1000) = 3100

FTE staffing requirements = 4.2

Weeks vacation offered = 5

Weeks vacation coverage required (5 weeks x 4.2 FTE) = 21 weeks

Additional FTE for vacation coverage (21 weeks/52 weeks) =
  0.4 additional FTE

Total FTE Coverage = 4.6 (round up to 5)

In the example cited above, three physicians would provide coverage for an average patient census of 45. Each hospitalist would be available for on-call duty every third or fourth night. To provide adequate physician coverage for on-call availability, the national average for cumulative annual in-hospital and out-of-hospital physician hours are applied to determine the total hours per physician FTE. If vacation is offered as an employee benefit, then additional physician FTEs will be required to cover this time. If additional FTEs are not provided for coverage of vacation time and the hospitalists are expected to cover each other's vacation, then vacation is not truly offered.

Shift-based model

The popularity of the shift-based model has increased as the number of hospitalist opportunities nationwide has increased. Hospitalists prefer this model because it provides for a better lifestyle. The model resembles the ED staffing model—24-hour in-house physician availability that is commonly divided into 12-hour shifts. Traditionally, these shift-based models incorporate a block schedule where staff physicians work continuous days followed by a number of days off. Ideally, the block stretch will be greater than the average patient length of stay to ensure continuity of care. In this model, most patients will be seen by the same physician throughout their hospital stay.

The most popular variations of this model include a seven days on/seven days off or five days on/five days off schedule. Hospitalists who follow this model may be scheduled for 14 or 15 shifts a month. Critics of this model consider it a part-time schedule. However, physicians who follow the shift-based model are clinically active for 180 hours a month, or 2160 hours a year—60 more hours than the standard work week of 40 hours.

The individual physician's stamina should determine the ideal length of each shift. Hospitalist programs that implement this model should also consider the possible disruption in the continuity of care that could result from one hospitalist ending his or her block shift as another hospitalist begins. To overcome this challenge, groups may opt to incorporate an "overlap" day. On the overlap day, the two hospitalists transitioning the service are both present. See **Figure 6.1.**

FIGURE **6.1** ILLUSTRATION OF 24-HOUR IN-HOUSE SHIFT BLOCK SCHEDULE UTILIZING SIX FTE

Week	Monday	Tuesday	Wednesday	Thursday	Friday	Saturday	Sunday
1		**AC**	**AC**	**AC**	**AC**	**ABC**	**BCD**
		E	E	E	E	E	F
2	**BD**	**BD**	**BD**	**BAD**	**ADE**	**AE**	**AE**
	F	F	F	F	C	C	C
3	**AE**	**ABE**	**BFE**	**BF**	**BF**	**BF**	**BCF**
	C	C	D	D	D	D	D
4	**CFE**	**CE**	**CE**	**CE**	**CED**	**EDF**	**DF**
	A	A	A	A	A	B	B
5	**DF**	**DF**	**DCF**	**FAC**	**AC**	**AC**	**AC**
	B	B	B	E	E	E	E
6	**ACD**	**ADB**	**DB**	**DB**	**DB**	**DBE**	**BAE**
	E	F	F	F	F	F	C
7	**AE**	**AE**	**AE**	**AEF**	**ABF**	**BF**	**BF**
	C	C	C	C	D	D	D
8	**BF**	**BFE**	**BCE**	**CE**	**CE**	**CE**	**CEF**
	D	D	A	A	A	A	A

The schedule alternates two teams of three physicians. Team one comprises physicians A, B, and C. Team two comprises physicians D, E, and F. Two physicians work during the daytime shifts, which are in bold type. Only one physician works during the night shifts. Physicians work in rotation—six day shifts are followed by five night shifts. Overlap days occur when three physicians are scheduled for a day shift. The physician going off duty will hand his or her patients off to the physician coming on duty. For example, in the block schedule, physician A is handing off patients to physician B on Saturday of week one.

Use the following calculation to determine the number of FTE needed to provide 24-hour physician staffing for a patient census of 45 for the sample schedule above:

ADC = 45

Ideal patient/physician load = 15

Daily rounding physicians = 3

Daily hours of in-house physician time

  (Night coverage + day coverage) = 48

  Day coverage (3 physicians x 12 hours) = 36

Night coverage (1 physician x12 hours) = 12

Hours per year physician time (48 hours x 365 days) = 17,520

Hours/FTE = 2100

FTE staffing requirements 17500 annual hours/ (2100 hours/FTE) = 8.3

Weeks vacation offered = 5

Weeks vacation coverage required (5 weeks x 8.3 FTE) = 42 weeks

Additional FTE for vacation coverage

  (42 weeks/52 weeks) = 0.8 additional FTE

Total FTE coverage = 9.1

As shown above, the 24-hour in-house model requires additional physician FTEs. For many large hospitalist programs, night volume may sustain night physicians' salaries. For smaller programs, the indirect value of providing 24-hour in-house physician availability may be best realized though the additional services it provides—real-time admitting, preoperative clearance medical consultation, night admitting service open to the medical staff, and code blue and emergency consult coverage.

Each model has advantages and disadvantages. The traditional call model allows maximum resource utilization and financial return. The shift-based model provides for ease of recruitment and sustainability. It is possible that programs that provide 24-hour in-house physician services may soon have quality implications similar to those of intensivists in the Leapfrog Group initiative (go to *www.leapfroggroup.org* for more information.)

As the hospitalist employment has increased and the demand for these physicians exceeds available resources, many new programs are turning away from call-based models and moving toward shift-based models as a recruitment tool. However, little is known about the sustainability of these staffing models in regard to career satisfaction and attrition. But many hospitalists, when faced with the option of choosing a traditional call model or a shift model, lean towards a shift based model for sustainability.

Vacation time

As demonstrated in the above examples, hospitalists programs must consider vacation time when determining staffing needs. Although the 2002 National Association of Inpatient Physicians benchmark survey indicated an average of six weeks of vacation, there is no data stratifying by staffing model. Do hospitalists practicing in call-based models have six weeks of vacation while those in shift based have none? Do nonscheduled days on a shift-based calendar count as vacation time? Unfortunately there is no data available on this topic. However, market pressures and aggressive hospitalist recruitment measures have created shift based programs that provide generous vacation packages in addition to "off-shift" time.

Professional satisfaction and the work environment

Beyond caseload and work hours, hospitalists' professional satisfaction is another item cited as a leading cause of attrition in established hospital medicine programs. Dissatisfied hospitalists complain of being treated like a resident. It's important for hospitalist programs to establish its goals up front to keep expectations aligned and resources secure. Hospitalists must decide whether the program will serve the call of the medical staff or clearly define the services it will offer. It must also determine whether PCPs who use hospitalists can select the patients they refer to the program. Keep in mind that the hospitalist group's employment model will influence the services it offers. Hospitalists employed by the hospital may be expected to admit all unassigned patients. However, hospitalists in private practice may only admit the unassigned patients for private physicians with whom they have established admitting relationships.

Professional satisfaction is as individualized as hospitalists themselves. However, the hospitalist program should ensure that its goals are aligned with the hospitalist's career goals. Aligning these goals will help prevent physician attrition and reduce recruitment costs.

Resources

Lurie, J.D., D.P. Miller, P.K. Lindenauer, R.M. Wachter, and H.S. Sox, "The potential size of the hospitalist workforce in the United States," *American Journal of Medicine.* 1999, 106, 441–5.

2002 National Association of Inpatient Physician Benchmark and Compensation Survey, www.hospitalmedicine.org.

Information Management to Assess Efficiency and Quality of Care

Patricia M. Gorman, RN, MSM, CPHQ

Information management is vital to the development and growth of a hospitalist program. These systems provide necessary information regarding the efficiency and quality of care delivered by hospitalists—information that is crucial to the group's success. However, many hospitalists struggle to initiate and maintain such systems.

To implement effective information management systems, the hospitalist group must first identify and define the value of quality and efficiency data to stakeholders. Hospital administrators are the key stakeholders in many hospitalist models. The establishment of mutually defined outcome goals is important to the hospitalist program and the institution since both require a means to measure the benefits delivered by the hospitalists.

The next step is to determine what to measure. This determination should be focused on the goals of the hospitalist program, as well as the economic and quality issues that affect the hospital. The hospital's quality management department, information services, administration, and the hospitalist director should be involved in this process. These key stakeholders should provide information that helps define mutual goals and should also explore current data collection and management systems.

Data collection

The hospital's information systems and those responsible for collecting the data play important roles in this process.

Hospital information systems

Hospitals have many databases to satisfy many different needs. Most organizations can generate quality and financial information from admission, discharge, and transfer databases. Financial information is often obtained from billing resources.

When designing information systems to measure hospitalists' performance, the group should consult the quality management, accounting, and medical records departments. In addition, hospitalists should examine the hospital's utilization review and case management information. For example, many hospitals use a MIDAS database. This system, which is similar to many other database systems, supports the utilization review process and collects useful data—including financial information. These databases contain relevant clinical data. Hospitalists should contact the hospital's utilization review, case management, or information systems departments for information about such databases.

Data collectors

Data collection is best done concurrently by people who understand the data definitions and are already doing chart review—typically members of the quality, case, or utilization management departments. These professionals often have a nursing background with clinical experience. In some facilities, the medical records department supports the chart review function. For data integrity and review of the charts, these departments have the people and the understanding to support data collection. Hospitalists must obtain support from these departments to collect program-specific data.

Hospitalists must understand who is collecting the data, how it is obtained, and where it is stored. The hospitalist program must secure the necessary resources to competently extract data from hospital databases to ensure the accuracy and validity of the information. Members from the hospitalist program should be involved in this process and develop expertise in data collection.

Determine what data to collect

Although the quantity of valuable data is limitless, hospitalists must focus on a relatively small fraction of this data to ensure efficient information management systems. Each hospitalist program must determine the appropriate data to collect and how much of that data to analyze. However, there are some generally accepted industry benchmarks that can guide this process. Most of the data currently collected by hospitalists is associated with efficiency, but the importance of quality data continues to increase.

Hospitalist programs often collect the following efficiency data:

- Patient volume

- Average age

- Length of stay—this data typically address overall lengths of stay, but may also be broken down into the top 10 or 20 diagnosis-related groups (DRGs) managed by the hospitalists

- Readmission rates

- Mortality

- Discharge disposition

- Charges/costs—this data is often broken down by DRG

Many hospitals and hospitalists currently use the Joint Commission on Accreditation of Health Care Organizations' core measurements as a guide (*go to www.jcaho.org/pms/core+measures/core+measures.htm*).

These measurements include the following:

- Acute myocardial infarction

- Aspirin prescribed on admission and at discharge

- Angiotension converting enzyme inhibitor for left ventricular dysfunction (ejection function < 40%)

- Beta-blocker on admission and at discharge

- Time to thrombolysis or percutaneous transluminal coronary angioplasty

- Smoking-cessation counseling

- Congestive heart failure

- Smoking cessation counseling

- Discharge instructions

- Community acquired pneumonia

Hospitalists might also consider the quality measures set forth by the Leapfrog Group (*www.leapfroggroup.org*). The Leapfrog Group's criteria include giving preference to organizations with high-volumes for certain procedures, computerized physician order entry, and to those organizations that meet intensivist staffing requirements for critical care units.

Hospitalists may also consult the new hospital requirements proposed by the National Quality Forum (*www.qualityforum.org*).

As each measure is selected, it is important that the definition of the measure is also determined. Although many of the measures mentioned above have standard definitions, some are open to local definition and interpretation. Stakeholders must understand and commit to the definition for the measure to have value. In addition, organizations that spend time collaborating and discussing the selection of information will reduce the time and frustration of implementing a data collection process.

Keep in mind that the population parameters must be addressed before the appropriate data is collected. Stakeholders must decide whether they only want data about acute inpatients, whether data about observation patients should be included, and whether readmission rates are important.

The type of patient hospitalists care for is important to the integrity of the data. This information is crucial when comparing hospitalists' performance against other practitioners' performance. For example, the maternal/child service population should not be included in the total patient count if hospitalists only treat acute medical-surgical patients over the age of 17.

Once the population is determined, time frames for measurement and data display can be discussed. Data integrity is essential. To avoid the "garbage in, garbage out" discussion, the data must be understood, defined, and protected. Though the case management or quality management department typically assesses the integrity of data, hospitalist program representatives must understand this process and monitor it closely.

Benchmarks and hospitalist program assessment

Once the stakeholders determine what data to collect, hospitalists must collect benchmarks against which they can compare their performance. There are two approaches to this issue in regard to efficiency measures. If the hospital has a sophisticated data collection and tracking system, it may be able to track non-hospitalist primary care physicians' (PCP) data as the control or comparison group.

This is the ideal method of comparison since the data represents the local standards the hospitalist program is striving to improve. In the absence of local comparison data, hospitalist programs may compare themselves to the Centers for Medicare & Medicaid Services' benchmarks.

Once efficiency and quality data is acquired, hospitalist programs should develop a process to systematically evaluate and assess the data. Though reviewing program data as a whole is crucial, programs should also evaluate each individual hospitalist's performance. Looking at individual performance allows for collaboration and healthy competition.

Remember: Once goals and measures are established, hospitalists must track indicators and consistently share this information with the group. These data are typically shared with physicians on a monthly, quarterly, or biannual basis. Consider presenting physicians with a profile of overall service and then discuss individual performance measures. Displaying the information in a graphic format with targets and benchmark data provides the opportunity to focus on improvement. It is important to have someone in attendance at the meeting who is familiar with the data, how it was collected, and how to interpret the information appropriately.

Keep in mind that the medical records department can provide important education and information about the coding process, principle diagnosis, principle procedure, and final DRG. This information can help answer hospitalists' questions about patient population and other data included on the profile. The medical records department can also help isolate data that applies to the hospitalist population if a database collection system is not available.

Implementing data collection systems

The absence of data presents obstacles when implementing data collection systems. The accuracy, appropriateness, and meaning of the data are often the subject of heated debate in these earlier stages. It's important that data-sharing sessions should focus on the goals that hospital and hospitalists hope to achieve by collecting the data, especially when the individual physicians are defensive about the information.

As the hospitalist program's patient volume increases, the data can be examined from different perspectives. In the early stages, the data should provide the hospitalist group with an overall picture of the program's patient volume, length of stay, mortality rate, readmission rate, and average patient. When a computer database for data collection is available, this information should be benchmarked against the hospitalists and then against the PCPs who treat the same patient population.

After the first six months of operation, the hospitalist program should have enough volume to support DRG comparison. Depending on volume, the top 10 or 15 hospitalist DRGs should be trended. The hospitalists should compare and drill down the data to improve performance. The data should pinpoint the processes in need of improvement. Hospitalists should then analyze the relevant medical records to determine how to best implement improvements.

Customer service

Customer service is an important component of quality improvement. Before hospitalists can obtain feedback from customers, they must first define the "customer" (see **Chapter 4** for more information). Patients are important customers of the hospitalist program The hospitalist group should determine whether the hospital has a customer service program. If so, the information collected by the hospital's program can be used to rank hospitalists' performance. This ranking allows hospitalists to improve the areas that patients value (see **Chapter 3** for more information).

Physicians who refer patients to the hospitalist group are also valuable customers. Feedback from the PCP regarding the hospitalist's care of his or her patient is important to maintaining these relationships. It is also important to track the top referring physicians. Hospitalists should contact patients and PCPs following the patient's discharge to collect additional data for improving the patient care process (see **Chapter 8** for more information about this topic).

Additional data sources

Increasing patient volume at many hospitals has led to overcrowded emergency departments (EDs) and a shortage of acute care beds. Surgery and other specialty procedures are occasionally postponed or cancelled because of hospital overcrowding. However, by quickly treating ED patients, the hospitalist can assess the appropriateness of an admission, determine the right level of care, and expedite admission. In addition, the hospitalists may discharge a subset of patients who would otherwise be admitted. It is important for hospitalists to have a mechanism to track these encounters.

At the other end of the spectrum, hospitalists can track an established target discharge to make more inpatient beds available and reduce lengths of stay. The discharge time should be measured by group and the individual hospitalist. The organization's admission, discharge, and transfer system allows it to compare overall discharge times against the hospitalists' rate.

The appropriateness of observation status v. inpatient admission is another indicator that hospitalists should track. The observation status demands early diagnosis and intervention. Since hospitalists provide continuous coverage, potential avoidable admissions and discharge delays can also be measured.

Hospitalists can track these indicators with relative ease and benchmark them against established standards.

Early ancillary referrals also help improve the ED process. A hospitalist can reduce the patient's length of stay by initiating ancillary assessments early in the care process. Tracking the use of ancillary services may demonstrate the value of the hospitalist program.

Hospitalists have the unique opportunity to influence the standardization of practice by developing clinical pathways and order sets. It is important for hospitalists to monitor compliance with these pathways—it will allow them to improve these care processes when patient variation occurs.

In addition, hospitalists' involvement in the development of and compliance with pathways and order sets can help reduce the average length of stay.

Keep in mind that the opportunity to collect data regarding cost-per-patient by DRG increases the value of variation-controlled care processes. The organization's accounting program is the best way to measure this value. If this type of program is unavailable, average charges v. average reimbursement can be used to create a baseline comparison. Support measurements should compare an individual hospitalist's use of the pathway with the average length of stay for that patient population.

Data collection process

A hospitalist report card can be developed using a database that captures specific performance data. The report card should include the hospitalist's name, whether he or she was the attending or consulting physician, when he or she first assessed the patient, and the referring physician's name. The report card should allow hospitalists to compare their performance to other attending physicians and against established benchmarks. A hospitalist report card is necessary and valuable to stakeholders, as it clearly displays meaningful outcomes data.

In addition to using information collected by databases, hospitalists can use the following methods to collect quality and efficiency data:

- **Concurrent or retrospective data collection**
  Keep in mind that concurrent or retrospective data collection is resource-intensive. The amount of data collected depends on the amount of dedicated resources. Before such data collection begins, hospitalists must decide what data elements to collect, which will determine the volume of charts that must be reviewed. The resources that hospitalists dedicate to this task will determine how best to collect the data. For example, discharge data can be collected using a "snapshot" approach. The snapshot approach looks at data collected during a specified time frame and makes assumptions about that information. If discharge times for all hospitalists is measured for one week, the assumption is that the discharge time is relatively stable.

• **Sample size collection**

Core quality measures can be calculated using sample-size collection. Hospitalists may choose to examine 30 cases or 5% of cases, whichever is larger, to produce a sample of the hospitalist group's practices.

• **Outcome measurement**

Outcome measurement requires hospitalists to dedicate a significant amount of resources. A daily review of new admissions, discharges, and continued stay patients would provide hospitalists with information regarding volume, mortality rates, average age, readmissions, and lengths of stay. This information could then be imported into a Microsoft Excel spreadsheet to produce a readable report.

Hospitalists must establish a process to determine the patient population. Again, this information can be obtained by using the organization's admission, discharge, and transfer systems.

Hospitalist programs must strive to constantly improve the quality patient care delivered at the hospital. It's essential for hospitalists to implement systems that attest to the quality of the program or they are of little value to the hospital.

According to the JCAHO's 2001 definition of quality, hospitalist programs must improve the following:

- **Efficacy**—The degree to which care has been shown to accomplish the desired out comes

- **Availability**—The degree to which appropriate care is made accessible to meet the patient/family needs

- **Optimality**—Ensuring the most advantageous balance between benefits and costs of care delivery and service

- **Timeliness**—Ensuring that care is provided with no delay and when needed

- **Continuity**—The degree to which care activities and services are coordinated among providers, settings and over time

- **Safety**—The degree to which the risk of an intervention or care environment is reduced for patients and providers

- **Respect and caring**—Providing care with sensitivity and respect for the patients' values, beliefs, expectations, and culture.

References

Cesta, Toni. G., A. Hussein, *The Case Manager's Survival Guide: Winning Strategies for Clinical Practice.* Tahan, Mosby, Inc. 2003

Center for Medicare & Medicaid Services Web Site. *http://cms.hhs.gov.*

Flary, Dominick L. and Suzanne Smith Blancett, *Handbook of Nursing Case Management: Health Care Delivery in a World of Managed Care.* Aspen Publishers, 1996.

Second-Generation Hospitalist Programs: Strategies for Securing Program Returns. Clinical Advisory Board, Washington, DC 2002.

The Comparative Performance of U. S. Hospitals The Source Book. Solucient, LLC, 2003

ORIENTATION AND MENTORING

MARY JO GORMAN, MD, MBA

DOTTIE PRICE

In the past, hospitalists' training and orientation have been processes of trial and error. However, the experiences of established hospitalist groups have identified several essential elements for starting and maintaining a successful hospitalist program.

Orientation is one such element. All hospitalist programs should make orientation a standard operating procedure. Orientation provides hospitalists and the practice group with a solid skill foundation and develops shared operational expectations. A well-constructed orientation process prepares hospitalists joining the practice group to provide appropriate care. Practice groups that simply welcome the new physician and then leave him or her stranded with minimal assistance are asking for disaster. Handing a new physician a pager and instructing him or her to simply go see some patients will not build or sustain a hospitalist practice.

In addition to orientation, mentoring plays an important role in a hospitalist group's success. Why bother mentoring hospitalists? After identifying and hiring candidates, an appropriate transition into their roles and the practice is critical to ensuring a solid, successful organization with a stable work force. Because success as a hospitalist requires skills that are not covered in residency programs, a structured approach to orientation and training is critical. All medical practices struggle to successfully train and orient a newly hired physician to the practice group. However, this challenge is especially difficult for hospitalists, which is an emerging specialty. But hospitalist groups that fail to successfully transition new practitioners risk attrition and employee dissatisfaction.

Begin the orientation and mentoring process

When considering a mentoring program for young hospitalists, it is important to set expectations. Begin by articulating the practice's expectations, norms, physician development goals, and strategy. It's also important to determine how much time is necessary to successfully orient physicians, and then sticking to that time frame even when incumbent physicians and the management team are tempted to short-circuit the program.

ORIENTATION AND MENTORING

The initial orientation for a physician entering a hospitalist practice should be four or five days, and never less than three. This plan eases new hires into practice by gradually increasing their responsibilities. An experienced hospitalist may be ready to assume the role in three days, but physicians transitioning from a residency program typically require four or five days of orientation.

The group may opt to continue the orientation process beyond the first stage by providing teaching modules over a longer period of time.

Set up the program

Take the following 10 steps to get your orientation program off the ground:

1. **Explain your practice model. Identify key operating principles and structures, and identify "deal-breaker" expectations for physicians practicing in your group.**

   Ask incumbent physicians to help the group determine the topics the orientation program should address. Sample topics include the following:

   • Practice structure and relationships

   • Workload expectations

   • Compensation plan design

- Schedule and call loop design

- Report and sign-out process

- Billing and coding education

- Documentation standards

- Rounding techniques

- Communication standards (such as using a personal digital assistant)

- Process for patient follow-up and handoff to the primary care provider

- Practice development

- Practice management

Once these key principles, structures, and expectations are identified, begin thinking about how to deliver this information to the new hospitalist. Some issues should be addressed immediately—schedule, call loop, attire, etc.—and others can be discussed later in the orientation process. The orientation program should be designed to address the most important topics first, which will allow the group to deliver the information to new physicians in manageable increments.

2. Outline the information above and provide specifics details.

Keep the outlined information focused, simple, and relevant. Organize the topics as standalones that could be combined to meet a new hospitalist's needs. For example, design a learning module for billing and coding. Prioritize what information to include in the module and in what order to deliver that information. Gather information on the topic and determine what materials you can use from your own supply and what must be customized. Lastly, put together a preliminary schedule to guide the building and deployment of learning modules.

3. Build the materials.

Once the content is organized, decide the best method for presenting the module to the new hospitalist. This determination will drive the design of the educational program and guide the development of new content. To make this decision, consider the available modes of delivering the material, which include oral briefings, written materials, video presentations, and Internet learning sessions.

The group may opt to use several methods to deliver the information. In addition to those mentioned above, the group may ask the physician's mentor to deliver the material in a one-on-one setting, develop self-study modules, or instruct the physician to participate in self-directed study on the Internet. Keep in mind that many adults learn by doing and will absorb content that is interesting to them. Design your program for relevance, ease of use, and scalability as the practice grows.

Consider how best to ensure that the new hospitalist absorbs the information. Information is best delivered in manageable doses and repeated in several places. Key concepts should be introduced, explained, and reinforced.

Remember that three-ring binders filled with orientation information tend to go unread. When possible, use facilitators to augment any written material to ensure physicians understand the information. If orientation materials are put into binders, the group should brief physicians about the information in the binder so they know where to go to look up information. Better yet, give physicians a number to call when they have questions after reviewing the material.

4. Pilot the materials on veteran doctors.

Before the group rolls out the orientation program, it should ask veteran doctors to test drive it to ensure

- the program captures the essence of the necessary operational detail, expectations, education material, etc.

- the content is relevant and accurately describes the hospitalist's role

- the defined priorities for information delivery are valid

- the physician's support for the program

The group's existing hospitalists who pilot the material are qualified to teach and reinforce the orientation information. Most practices begin with a lot of unwritten history and business process. Few groups take the time to standardize their operations. The group should ensure that the orientation program accurately reflects the group's current practices so that new hires aren't be taught tactics and expectations that veteran physicians don't know about. It is critical that the new hospitalist and the incumbents both know the organization's standard procedures and expectations.

Disorganized hospitalist practices can begin to restructure by following the steps outlined above. Engage veteran physicians by articulating desired operational details, obtaining their buy-in for the emerging strategy, and discussing how to transition new hospitalists.

5. Identify a well-matched physician mentor.

It is critical that new hospitalists are appropriately matched with a mentor who will assist them during transition. A peer mentor should be carefully selected since he or she will help determine the overall success of the orientation experience.

During the interview and selection process, the hospitalist practice should gather information about the candidate that will help it match him or her with a mentor with a similar personality and background. Occasionally, the group will be forced to pair a new hospitalist with a less-than-ideal mentor. In such situations, program staff or the program manager should schedule additional activities to ensure the new physician's questions are being answered, orientation is proceeding, and he or she is being supported.

Develop a set of criteria to qualify physicians as mentors and match your physicians against these criteria. In some instances, the group will add physicians more quickly than it can add mentors. As previously discussed, groups that select weak mentors should provide new hospitalists with additional support.

A good peer mentor should

- be a solid role model in the areas that were identified as critical to the practice's success and stability: communication, rounding efficiency, relationships with others, clinical excellence, and quality

- have the time necessary to assist and support the new hospitalist

- have an interest in teaching

- support the practice's culture

It's important for hospitalist groups to determine the time commitment peer mentors must make to effectively orient new hospitalists. To make this determination, divide the peer mentors into two categories: resource doctor (RD) and practice partner (PP). The RD is not a member of the practice the new physician will join. However, the PP is a member of the practice. These roles are defined as follows:

- The RD functions as the hospitalist's role model and demonstrates essential hospitalist skills to new hospitalists in a clinical setting. For a portion of the first week of orientation, the new hire should be scheduled to shadow the RD during his or her daily routine. The experience is less about clinical medicine and more about the RD setting expectations and demonstrating work habits, efficiency, and relationship building. Again, the RD is not in the same practice as the new physician. A neutral party outside the practice provides the new physician with a mentor in whom he or she can confide. The RD also exposes the new hospitalist to other styles of organizing the work process.

- The PP shows the new hire the day-to-day operational ropes, including the political lay of the land, where to park, who to know, consultation patterns, etc. This physician mentor is in the same practice and preferably practices at the same hospital as the new physician.

  The PP model allows physicians in the practice to teach while limiting the strain the orientation process has on their time.

6. Train physician mentors.

It is important to train the mentors who will teach new hospitalists. Hospitalist groups should provide physician mentor candidates and train them how to interact with new hires. In addition, senior physicians should reinforce the group's expectations for the orientation process to ensure a cohesive work group.

The quality of the practice's performance increases when both the mentor and new hospitalists are trained on the key topics discussed above. True mentors usually take to this role with zeal and learn the content so they can teach effectively. Even those mentors who participate in the orientation process with little enthusiasm will understand the need for a standard approach, especially in a busy practice where problems disrupt the practice and creates issues for all partners. Most physicians welcome processes that set practice norms and expectations that may have gone undocumented in the past.

7. **Develop a schedule for accomplishing orientation program activities, and train administrative staff in the basics of the program.**
No practice can afford to have new physicians in training indefinitely. The orientation schedule must be designed, implemented, and supported to ensure key topics are consistently covered. Practices are often busy and assert that they cannot spare time to educate new hospitalists. However, hospitalist groups must have the discipline to maintain the training schedule even when short-term adjustments have to be made.

For example, a group may distribute orientation materials during the first week and schedule two-hour learning modules for the next six or seven weeks. The group must allow some leeway to postpone these modules when there are significant time constraints. The orientation process must build-in flexibility to accommodate operational reality.

Lastly, the group should train its administrative staff about the basics of the orientation system since they will help support the program by ensuring that the new physician schedules and completes the topics. This education will help the program function and relieve physicians of administrative duties.

8. Provide program support for deployment, monitoring and improvement.

The group should assign accountability and responsibility for the orientation program and the new hospitalists to a program manager. The program manager should have a clinical background with the ability to juggle administrative responsibilities and complex project management tasks. The program manager should collaborate with physicians when required, and run the day-to-day operations of the orientation program. The group's executive assistant may also support orientation activities.

New physicians often appreciate having a contact person beyond the practice group who is committed to their success. Depending on the scope and depth of the program, this contact can be either an administrative person or a lead physician. In either case, the program must be supported, actively monitored, and revised when things don't go as planned. The group should build this infrastructure with the same care as the program content. Appropriate assignment of responsibility and accountability is essential to sustaining the orientation program.

Finally, it is critical for practice partners to understand and support mentors and new hospitalists by helping distribute the patient care work on the days identified for training.

9. Build follow-up and feedback loops into the program.

Program evaluations must ensure viability and relevance. The hospitalist group should track how long it takes to complete each training module, and ask new physicians to evaluate the content, relevance, and performance of the facilitator. New physicians should also rate the training program's overall value.

This feedback may trigger the implementation of additional educational programs offered to the group's entire physician work force. In addition, the feedback should be used when reviewing and revising the orientation program, and incorporated into the evaluation of program mentors.

10. Complete the process with a final review.

The supervising physicians should conduct of a full evaluation of the hospitalist at the conclusion of the formal orientation process. A site visit provides the supervising physician an opportunity to see how well the new hospitalist has adjusted to his or her role, ask for feedback about the overall orientation program, and provide direct education and follow-up on issues noted during the one-on-one visit.

The supervising physician should review the following topics with the new hospitalist:

- Quality of clinical notes

- Relationships within the hospital

- Work habits and rounding efficiency

- Medical record completion

- Resource utilization

- Relationships with local practice partners and management

The orientation overview should discuss the site visit to ensure new hospitalists are not surprised at the end of the orientation process. Hospitalists who are prepared for the visit often welcome the opportunity to meet one-on-one with a senior physician. After making rounds with the new hospitalist, the supervising physician can ask the hospitalist how he or she is adjusting, what they feel is working well, what frustrates them, and how they are handling the workload.

The group should develop a template to guide the site visit. The group should note the observations made by supervising physician during the site visit, as well as the new hire's feedback, and provide any necessary follow-up.

It takes a great deal of time and energy to develop an effective orientation program—resources that a small hospitalist program may lack. In such situations, the program should focus on implementing the following elements:

- Explain the practice model and expectations. Once this information is identified, members of the group should review it with the hospitalist candidate before he or she provides patient care. Set aside time for the new physician to study the information.

- Schedule regular group meetings. Conduct these meetings at least monthly. Weekly meetings are ideal.

- Identify someone who can train your physicians on billing and coding practices. Make this training mandatory for all new physicians.

Hospitalist medicine is rapidly becoming not just a model for inpatient care, but the dominant model. Those who succeed in this specialty will define the necessary skill set, hire new physicians based on those skills, and help develop hospitalists' skills through their tenure with the practice.

FINANCIAL OPERATIONS

WAYNE O. WINNEY, MHA, CMPE

The financial elements of a hospitalist program are often the most difficult to assess. However, an accurate assessment of a hospitalist program's costs and billing services is essential to its success.

Assessing costs

Costs are generally divided into three categories: direct, indirect, and capital. Direct costs include hospitalists' salaries and benefits. Typical indirect costs include nonphysician personnel, including nurses and case managers. Indirect costs may also include billing service expenses and office space. Capital costs, which include items such as cell phones, computers, and fax machines, are usually minimal for a hospitalist program.

According to a recent National Association of Inpatient Physicians (now the Society of Hospital Medicine) compensation and productivity survey, the median hospitalist program overhead was 20%, though there was much variability in this estimate. Keep in mind that the hospitalist group's relationship with a group practice or hospital will determine the expense structure. However, generally speaking, the hospitalist should have limited overhead amounts or costs.

Physician compensation

Physician compensation is often a hospitalist programs' largest expense. Remember that compensation is affected by the nature of the program and the economic environment in which it exists. The four basic types of compensation available to hospitalists include:

- **Productivity**

  The productivity model compensates the physician on net receipts less expenses. For the purpose of this example, net receipts are gross receipts (cash received) less expenses. Expenses are those that are directly related to the physician, and include taxes—Federal Insurance Compensation Act, retirement/pension plan contributions, continuing medical education (CME) and travel expenses, books, publications, professional dues, medical education, malpractice insurance, health insurance, disability insurance, life insurance, cost of administrative personnel, and office space rent.

Productivity compensation encourages the hospitalist to work more to earn more. However, there are several disadvantages to this model. The incentive for the physician to work harder is based on receipts, which is driven by payer type. The payer mix encountered by a program could significantly affect the hospitalist's ability to meet income goals. In addition, for a team of hospitalists, this could create problems with patient selection bias/avoidance by payer type.

For example, commercial payers reimburse inpatient services at approximately 80% of charges, and Medicare and Medicaid reimburse at approximately 50%. It is easy to see that, under productivity-based compensation, physicians may start considering what type of payers they want to treat. In addition, this type of compensation offers no incentives for efficiency—an important factor in the majority of hospitalist programs.

- **Salary plus bonus**

  Salary plus bonus is a common method of compensation for hospitalists. To determine the appropriate market rate for a hospitalist's salary, review the Medical Group Management Association's (MGMA) *Physician Compensation Survey* and the National Association of Inpatient Physicians' first *Compensation and Productivity Survey* mentioned above.

  In this model, benefits are a significant part of the compensation plan, both for the employee and the employer.

- **Combination**

  Organizations can take several different approaches to determine a combination bonus. However, the calculation should be kept as uncomplicated as possible. For example, many formulas use a percentage for overhead, which then sets the threshold for obtaining a bonus. If the hospitalist receives an annual salary of $150,000, the overhead, which contains all the benefits and the administrative costs for the practitioner, is 40%. Therefore, after the hospitalist generates revenue greater than salary and overhead combined, he or she is eligible for a bonus.

- **Salary with no bonus**

  Another approach to compensation is the accurate costs or expenses method. For example, the physician earns $150,000 annual salary and receives $55,000 in benefits and expenses. In some locations teaching may be an expectation. In such situations, compensation may be structured as a salary or stipend for teaching and salary plus bonus for clinical services.

If the hospitalist program decides to implement a bonus program, it must ensure that the program rewards teamwork in addition to individual performance. Incentive plans must make it clear to physicians that they can positively affect the program. To drive this point home to hospitalists, some groups use a hybrid bonus method that rewards the team for performance and individual hospitalists for productivity.

For example, if the hospitalist program is not covering its costs, no one in the group receives a bonus even if one or more physicians perform above the calculations set for bonuses. If the program is efficient and successful, all physicians are eligible for a bonus. Keep in mind that although this approach does reward the physicians for working well as a team, it may create disincentive for hardworking physicians if workloads are not equal among members of the group.

Vacation time and CME are also significant benefits that the hospitalist program should factor into its expenses. These benefits may be a direct expense if a program is on a shift-based system, or indirect if the physicians share call equally throughout the year and are expected to cover their full yearly amount of call. (See **Chapter 4** for a complete discussion of this issue.)

The mechanics of claims submission

Insurers require medical practices to collect and submit specific billing information following a strict format. Deviation from this format may cause the insurer to deny the payment request.

When submitting a claim to an insurer or payer, the practitioner must complete a form called a CMS 1500. The form includes 33 required entries that must be completed before the payer will process the claim. A missing or incomplete entry will usually result in a rejection from the payer, who will then return the bill unpaid.

Note: Although CMS 1500 forms can be printed and submitted by mail, most payers will accept these forms electronically. Most billing services now accept claims submitted electronically, and these services often provide remittance electronically. However, the Centers for Medicare & Medicaid Services (CMS) does require payers to follow a specific format for submitting electronic claims. Electronic billing and remittance requires secure information system, which may not be financially feasible for some facilities. Organizations that lack the funds to implement such systems may opt to outsource their billing services.

Incomplete claim forms returned to the organization must be corrected and resubmitted—delaying the payment process. The most effective billing services are able to submit clean claims that are promptly paid. Such services employ trained and experienced personnel and rely on modern information systems. Billing services are also increasingly turning to specialized software programs to evaluate claims for completeness before submission—a process known as "scrubbing." Incomplete claims are identified, completed, and then submitted—decreasing the number of rejected claims and increasing cash flow for the practice.

For example, CMS typically processes correctly submitted electronic claims within 10 to 14 days. When billing CMS electronically, the practice can track the status of that claim through CMS. This feature allows a billing operation to forecast the cash availability—a valuable tool for medical practices, which are sensitive to variations in cash. Electronic billing helps these practices manage such variations.

In addition, payers that provide electronic remittance can also electronically deposit payments into the practice's bank account and provide an electronic explanation and details of the payments received. Most billing services will recommend this approach for speed and convenience.

Quality and accounts receivable (AR)

Hospitalists should be familiar with the term, "days in AR," which refers to the time it takes to receive payment for a bill once it is submitted. This term can help hospitalists assess the quality of a billing service. For example, the following analogy can be used to guide the evaluation of billing services (please forgive the liberties taken from cardiology).

The sum amount of daily charges provides the basis for determining a practices' potential value in terms of actual revenue. The total charges can be considered the heart rate of the practice, which rises and falls, and represents the practice's potential revenue generation.

Next, consider the days in AR as the practice's blood pressure. The average days in AR for all practice charges are an indication of the health of the practice's receivable management. Thus, 40 days in AR is normal blood pressure. However, 80 or 90 days in AR indicates low blood pressure.

Lastly, the aging of ARs can be considered the organization's lipid profile. Hospitalists should require their billing service to provide them with reports regarding the aging of their ARs, which divides ARs into stratified time periods. According to the 2002 MGMA cost survey, the average distributions for internal medicine practices are as follows:

- Current (<30 days) = 44.50%

- 31–60 days = 16.68%

- 61–90 days = 8.57%

- 91–120 days = 5.03%

- >120 days = 21.51%

The above statistics are important for the physician to understand. The ratio of days in AR indicates the speed in which claims are turned into cash (blood pressure). The "aging" provides the description of the number of claims that are current as well as the number that are old. In general, claims that take longer than 180 days to process tend to be self-pay and will likely not be collectable.

A good mix, or lipid profile, in the distribution of the ages of ARs suggests the collections process is effective. It is also one of the main means for evaluating the billing service's performance.

The hospitalist group may want to provide the billing service with directions on when to send an account to a collection agency and when to write-off an account. The latter is an action that only the practice can decide to take and should not be left to the billing service to determine. Billing is a necessary part of conducting business. No matter how often it is said that physicians are not good businesspeople, physicians must understand and effectively interpret the statistics of its billing service.

Selecting a billing service

The effectiveness of an organization's billing process depends on the billing service it employs. When selecting a billing service, the group must first identify and interview several different potential vendors to ensure that it makes an educated decision. Keep the following tips in mind when evaluating a potential billing service:

- Gather recommendations from other medical practices that use the billing service. A testimonial from a trusted colleague who is satisfied with the service is valuable. The billing service should provide at least two references from hospitalist groups or inpatient practices with which it currently works.

- Pay attention to billing that the vendor has been involved with in the past. Can the service provide the billing services that practice needs? For example, a billing service that specializes in outpatient orthopedics or ophthalmology may not understand the nuances of inpatient billing.

- Determine whether the service submits the majority of bills electronically.

- Determine the average number of days in AR.

- Find out how many practices currently use the service and how many practices terminated their relationships with the service in the last year.

- Conduct the interview at the billing service's facilities. Meet the staff and have them explain how their service works. Make sure the staff has adequate time to work the practice's accounts.

- Find out how the service will report its performance to the practice.

Once a billing service is chosen, meet with its staff on a regular basis. Consider keeping minutes of issues or concerns discussed during these meetings to ensure follow-up. MGMA developed a checklist and questionnaire for its members that can be used to assess a billing service. Go to *www.mgma.com* for more information.

When entering into a contractual relationship with a billing service, ensure that the contract clearly defines the service it will provide. In addition, the contract should address the following:

- Notices and potential penalties

- Ownership of data and data formats

- Automatic contract extensions

- Written notice requirements

- Termination options

- Continuation beyond termination date

The practice group's attorney should review the contract. This additional cost may save the practice money in the long run.

Remember, a billing service is only effective when hospitalists provide complete, timely, and accurate charges to the service. Many physicians consider the billing side of clinical care a nuisance—one they would like to avoid all together. Therefore, physicians may submit illegible, incomplete, or old billing cards or documents to the billing department. Physicians must be reminded that their compliance with the billing process is essential for the practice's success.

The practice management must implement a process that makes billing as easy as possible. Consider designating a location for physicians to submit billing documents. The location should be a place physicians must pass during the day or just before leaving the hospital. The timely collection of these documents will reflect greatly on the days in AR and aging reports—and ultimately the financial viability and health of the hospitalist program.

References

Cleverly, William O. *Essentials of Health Care Finance, Second Edition.* Aspen Publication, Aspen Publishers, Inc. Gaithersberg, MD. 1986.

NAIP, *2002 Productivity and Compensation Survey (www.hospitalmedicine.org).*

MGMA, *Physician Compensation and Production Survey,* 2003 *Report Based on 2003 Data, www.mgma.com.*

Solomon, Robert J. *The Physician Manager's Handbook: Essential Business Skills for Succeeding in Healthcare.* Aspen Publication, Aspen Publishers, Inc. Gaithersberg, MD. 1997

CODING BASICS
FOR HOSPITALISTS

CHARLEEN PORTER, BS, MA, CPC

Physicians work in one of the most highly regulated business sectors in the United States. It is imperative that physicians have at least a basic understanding of procedural and diagnostic coding.

However, appropriately coding physician services may be one of the most frustrating and challenging task a physician must tackle, as his or her reimbursement may be directly related to how accurately he or she assigns codes to services rendered. But accurate codes may result in speedier claims payments and reduced chances for audit.

This chapter outlines the majority of evaluation and management (E/M) codes used by hospitalists, provides assistance for choosing the level of service, suggests necessary reference materials, and provides useful resources.

Importance of coding

Hospitalists must learn how to appropriately assign codes to avoid costly and time-consuming appeals and refunds to payers. In other words, hospitalists must learn this skill to ensure that they receive appropriate payment the first time. Keep in mind that inaccurate coding can results in far more serious actions than a refund request. The False Claims Act and other federal regulations may be used to prosecute physicians who use incorrect codes. Penalties include civil monetary penalties, exclusion from government programs, and incarceration.

Because of the numerous penalties a physician may incur if he or she uses incorrect codes, physicians often employ a coding expert to code and bill services. However, physicians who hire coding experts remain ultimately responsible for the accuracy of claims submitted to Medicare, Medicaid, and other insurers.

A coding consultant may also be helpful and does not have to be expensive. It is worthwhile for a physician to meet with a consultant annually to stay up-to-date with coding, billing, and policy changes that affect his or her practice.

Consult reference materials

At the minimum, every physician should have the current year's *Current Procedural Terminology* (commonly called the CPT book), HCPCS Level II

Codes, and ICD-9 CM (a book of diagnoses). The World Health Organization compiles both the ICD-9 CM and HCPCS Level II Codes. These resources, which are revised annually, are published by numerous companies.

CPT codes and ICD-9 codes are the language physicians use to describe the services they render to patients. The more physicians understand about how to use codes, the better they can communicate with those who pay them for services. If physicians want to get paid, they must learn to speak the language of insurers.

E/M services

MCM ∫15501 E/M service codes—general (codes 99201–99499),
Medical necessity of a service is the primary criterion for payment and for individual requirements of a CPT code. It is not medically necessary or appropriate to bill a higher level of E/M service when a lower level of a service is warranted. The level of service billed should not be based on the amount of documentation. Documentation should instead support the level of service reported. The service should be documented during or soon after the service is provided to ensure the accuracy of the medical record.

1. **CPT codes 99217–99220—Observation care services**
   CPT codes 99221–99239—Hospital inpatient services

   These series of codes are used to report E/M services rendered to observation patients and hospital inpatients that are not admitted and discharged on the same day unless they are inpatients or in observation for less than eight hours.

• The initial observation care codes (99218–99220) and initial hospital care codes (99221–99223) should be used to report the first encounter with the patient in the observation or inpatient setting.

• The observation and inpatient hospital descriptors contain the phrase "per day," which means that the code represents all services provided to the patient on that date, even if the services began in a different site of service, such as the emergency department (ED).

For example, physician A sees the patient in the morning and physician B (both of same group), who is covering for A, sees the same patient in the evening. Insurers will not pay physician B for the second visit. However, there is an exception to this rule. If physician B provides services that qualify as critical care services, both physician A and B may bill their services. Keep in mind that the reverse is not true. If the patient receives critical care services from physician A in the morning and physician B rounds on the patient in the evening, only physician A's charges will be considered for payment.

• When physicians are each responsible for a different aspect of the patient's care, Medicare will pay both visits if the physicians are in different specialties and the visits are billed with different diagnoses.

• Medicare will pay for an initial hospital care service or an initial inpatient consultation if a physician sees the patient in the ED and admits the patient.

• All services provided by the physician in conjunction with that admission are considered part of the initial hospital care when performed on the same date as the admission.

• Medicare will only pay the admission service—not a discharge service—when a patient is admitted either as observation status or an inpatient for less than eight hours on the same calendar date.

• When the patient is admitted and discharged on the same date of service and has remained an inpatient for at least eight hours or more, CPT codes 99234–99236 should be billed. These codes may be billed whether the patient is in observation status or admitted as an inpatient.

These codes are for admission and discharge services performed on the same date. The same codes represent admission and discharge for either inpatient or observation services. Medicare requires the patient be an inpatient or in observation for at least eight hours to use 99234–99236. Both the admission and the discharge must be documented. The physician must inform the billing department whether the patient is an inpatient or in observation. The billing department will not know the patient's status (inpatient v. observation) unless the physician shares this information.

• An initial hospital care code (admission) and a hospital discharge management code may be billed when the discharge and admission do not occur on the same date.

• If the same physician admits the patient to a hospital following a nursing facility visit on the same date, Medicare will pay only the initial hospital care code and will not pay a nursing facility visit.

References: *MCM* §15505.1—payment for initial hospital care services, and *MCM* §15505—payment for inpatient hospital visits

2. CPT codes 99217–99220—Hospital observation services

This series of codes is used to report services rendered to patients in an observation unit who are not admitted and discharged on the same day—unless they are in an observation for less than eight hours. The severity of the illness/intensity of services rendered must require institutional care for the services to be covered. Admission to an observation unit is appropriate when release from the hospital the same day or the next day can reasonably be expected.

There must be a medical observation record for the patient that contains the physician's admitting orders—dated and timed—regarding the care the patient is to receive while in observation. The record must also include nursing notes and progress notes prepared by the physician while the patient was in the observation unit. This record must be in addition to records prepared during an ED or outpatient clinic encounter.

• Medicare will only pay the initial observation care code when the patient is discharged on the same date he or she is admitted to observation and there for less than eight hours.

• When the patient is discharged on the same date he or she is admitted to observation and has been in observation for more than eight hours on the same calendar date, CPT codes 99234–99236 may be used to bill Medicare for these services. Both the admission service and the discharge service must be documented.

• If the patient remains in observation on the day after the date he or she is admitted to observation, the expectation is that the patient would be discharged on that second day. CPT code 99217 would be billed for observation care discharge services provided on the second date.

• If a patient is held in observation status for more than two calendar dates, the physician must bill subsequent services furnished before the date of discharge using the outpatient office visit codes (99212–99215).

• Medicare will only pay the inpatient admission service if the physician who admitted a patient to observation status also admits the patient to inpatient status before the end of the observation admission date.

• If the patient is admitted to inpatient status from observation, the physician must bill an initial hospital visit for the services provided on that date. The observation discharge code may not be billed.

Reference: *MCM* §15504—Payment for hospital observation services

3. CPT codes 99221–99223—Initial hospital care services

Medicare will pay for an initial hospital care service or initial inpatient consultation if the physician sees the patient in the ED and then admits him or her to the hospital. When the patient is admitted to the hospital via another site of service (e.g., hospital ED, physician's office, nursing facility), all services provided by the physician in conjunction with that admission are considered part of the initial hospital care when performed on the same date as the admission.

When the *Medicare Carrier's Manual* indicates either an initial hospital care service (admission) or an initial inpatient consultation may be billed, it is making a distinction between "initial" (99251–99255) and "follow-up" (99261–99263). A follow-up inpatient consultation code is used to complete the initial consultation or a subsequent consultative service requested by the attending physician.

• Medicare will pay for both visits when the patient is seen in the physician's office on one date and admitted to the hospital on the next date, even when less than 24 hours has elapsed between the visit and admission.

• Medicare will pay only the initial hospital care code when a patient is admitted as an inpatient and discharged on the same day. The system will not pay the hospital discharge management code on the date of admission.

• Medicare will only pay the admission service if the patient has been an inpatient for less than eight hours. Hospital discharge management will not be paid separately. A code that combines admission and discharge on the same day may be billed to Medicare if the patient has been an inpatient for more than eight hours on the same day. (See Same Date Admission and Discharge Services in the *MCM*.)

• Physicians may bill both the hospital discharge management code and an initial hospital care code when the discharge and admission do not occur on the same day if the transfer is between different hospitals, different facilities under common ownership that do not have merged records, or between the acute care hospital and a prospective payment system (PPS) exempt unit within the same hospital when there are no merged records.

• When a patient is admitted on one date and transferred on a subsequent date, a discharge management code may be billed, rather than a subsequent hospital visit code, if the patient is transferred to a different hospital, different facilities under common ownership that do not have merged records, or between the acute care hospital and a PPS-exempt unit within the same hospital when there are no merged records.

• In all other transfer circumstances, the physician should bill only the appropriate level of subsequent hospital care for the date of transfer.

• When the physician performs a visit or consultation that meets the definition of a level five office visit or consultation several days prior to an admission, and on the day of admission performs less than a comprehensive history and physical, he or she should report the office visit or consultation that reflects the services furnished. The physician should also report the lowest level initial hospital care code (i.e., 99221) for the initial hospital admission.

• The admitting physicians should use the initial hospital care codes (99221–99223) to report the first hospital inpatient encounter with the patient.

• Medicare will allow only one admitting physician, and only the admitting physician can use initial hospital care codes. If another physician participates in the care of a patient but is not the admitting physician of record, he or she should bill the inpatient E/M service codes that describe his or her participation in the patient's care (e.g., subsequent hospital visit, inpatient consultation).

• Medicare will pay only the initial hospital care code if the patient is admitted to a hospital following a nursing facility visit on the same date by the same physician. Physicians may not report a nursing facility service and an initial hospital care service on the same day. Payment for the initial hospital care service includes all work performed by the physician in all sites of service on that date.

Reference: *MCM* §15505.1—Payment for initial hospital care services

4. CPT codes 99231–99239—Subsequent hospital visit and hospital discharge management

Medicare will pay only the hospital discharge management code on the day of discharge (unless it is also the day of admission, in which case, the admission service and not the discharge management service is billed). Medicare will not pay both a subsequent hospital visit in addition to hospital discharge day management service on the same day by the same physician.

• Medicare will pay the hospital discharge code (99238 or 99239) in addition to a nursing facility admission code when billed by the same physician with the same date of service—as long as the physician sees the patient at both sites on the same date.

• If a surgeon is admitting the patient to the nursing facility due to a condition that is not as a result of the surgery during the postoperative period of a service with the global surgical period, he or she bills for the nursing facility admission and care with a -24 modifier and provides documentation that the service is unrelated to the surgery.

For example, the return of an elderly patient to the nursing facility in which he or she has resided for five years following discharge from the hospital.

• Medicare will not pay for a nursing facility admission in the postoperative period of a procedure with a global surgical period if the patient is admitted to the nursing facility for postoperative care related to the surgery (e.g., admission to a nursing facility to receive physical therapy following a hip replacement). Payment for the nursing facility admission and subsequent nursing facility services are included in the global fee and cannot be paid separately.

• The discharge day management codes 99238 or 99239 are time-based codes. When 99239 is billed, the physician's documentation must include the minutes spent discharging the patient. However, the time may be accumulated, not necessarily continuous. The documented time must include only physician time and may not include time spent by others involved in providing discharge services.

• The discharge day management codes include, "as appropriate, final examination of the patient, discussion of the hospital stay, even if the time spent by the physician on that date is not continuous, instructions for continuing care to all relevant caregivers, and preparation of discharge records, prescriptions and referral forms." These services are face-to-face services. Therefore, Medicare will not pay for discharge day management when the physician discharges the patient via telephone.

Reference: *MCM* §15505.2—Subsequent Hospital Visit and Hospital Discharge Management
Current Procedural Terminology CPT 2003, American Medical Association

5. CPT codes 99234–99236—Same date admission and discharge services

These codes are used to report observation or inpatient hospital care services provided to patients admitted and discharged on the same date of service. To use these codes for a Medicare patient, the patient must have been an inpatient or an observation care patient for a minimum of eight hours on the same calendar date.

• The physician must clearly indicate in the patient's medical record the hours the patient was in observation or inpatient status when billing CPT codes 99234–99236 to Medicare.

• The physician must satisfy the documentation requirements for both admission to and discharge from inpatient or observation care to bill CPT codes 99234, 99235, or 99236.

Reference: November 1, 2000 *Federal Register*, p. 65409

Transitional care services

Transitional or alternative care units have become commonplace in today's hospital environment. The beds may also be called "swing" beds, and are typically licensed by the Department of Health. The majority of these beds are certified as acute care hospital beds, nursing facility beds, or a mixture of the two.

The units that house swing beds have evolved, and care received in these beds may vary from advanced care to nursing home care. Patients in these beds are always considered inpatients. However, the certification of the bed determines the place of service and CPT codes used to bill services rendered in the bed. If the patient is billed by the hospital as inpatient care, then the inpatient place of service (21) and inpatient care codes (99221–99239) should be used to bill the services. If the patient is billed by the hospital as skilled nursing facility care, then the nursing facility place of service (31), and nursing facility codes (99301–99316) should be used to bill the services.

Reference: *MCM* §15505.D

The patient/hospitalist handoff: Choose the type of service

To assign appropriate codes, hospitalists must determine whether they are being asked to

- admit and follow the patient throughout their inpatient stay

- manage the patient's conditions unrelated to his or her admitting diagnosis
- evaluate or evaluate and treat a specific condition or aspect of the patient's care

- perform a preoperative evaluation of the patient

If the hospitalist is asked to admit the patient and follow him or her throughout the course care, the initial inpatient care codes and discharge service codes outlined above would be billed: 99218–99220 (initial observation care), 99217 (observation discharge), 99221–99223 (initial hospital care), 99231–99233 (subsequent hospital care), 99238–99239 (hospital discharge services, or 99234–99236 (observation or inpatient care services, including admission and discharge).

If the admitting physician asks the hospitalist to manage the patient's conditions unrelated to his or her admitting diagnosis, subsequent hospital care codes should be used to follow the patient's hospital stay. These codes would be 99231–99233 (subsequent hospital care).

For example, the patient is admitted with a hip fracture and the hospitalist is asked to manage the patient's diabetes or hypertension. This is not a consultative role. The hospitalist is not being asked for his or her opinion, but rather to assume care of the patient's conditions unrelated to the hip fracture. The level of visit will depend on the number and severity of the conditions the hospitalist actively treats or manages. In addition, the hospitalist should use only the diagnoses he or she is actively managing and not the diagnoses related to the patient's admission. This will help reduce concurrent care denials by insurers. However, if the patient's condition(s) are stable, an insurer may question the medical necessity of having the hospitalist follow the patient.

When the hospitalists is asked to evaluate or and treat a specific condition or aspect of the patient's care, he or she should determine whether

- the patient known to the inpatient physician/group

- the patient is known to the physician/group

- the physician has been following the patient for a specific condition, and if so, whether there has been a significant change in the patient's conditions since he or she was last seen by the inpatient physician/group

The answers to these questions are especially important because of the diversity within inpatient practices. Some physicians are solely hospital-based while others split their time between an inpatient practice and an office based practice.

A hospitalist who is asked to evaluate a patient with whom he or she is already familiar should not use a consultation code for the request to evaluate. The service should be billed with a subsequent care code, CPT 99231–99233. However, if it has been some time since the hospitalist has seen the patient, or if there has been a significant change in the patient's status, he or she should bill a consultation code.

The hospitalist should use a consultation code if asked to perform a preoperative evaluation of the patient. Remember, Medicare may consider a preoperative service, performed in the absence of signs or symptoms, a routine service and deny the consultation for lack of medical necessity. In addition, for Medicare purposes, the preoperative diagnosis should be the first diagnosis coded, the reason for the surgery (e.g., knee replacement, cataract, etc.) should be the second diagnosis, and the third diagnosis should reflect current or active signs, symptoms, or conditions.

Determine the level of service

The following paragraphs and illustrations include highlights of the *Documentation Guidelines for E/M Services*. Keep in mind that this information does not represent the guidelines in their entirety. There are numerous clarifications contained in the guidelines that are not included here. To reference the complete *Documentation Guidelines for E/M Services* go to *www.cms.hhs.gov.*

These guidelines were intended to be used by auditors and are not designed to be used by physicians to determine a level of service prior to billing the service to Medicare or other insurers.

However, the guidelines provide physicians with insight into how services are reviewed and audited. Physicians should use this information to help choose a level of service. Ideally, the physician should use the *Documentation Guidelines for E/M Services* to work though examples of his or her own documentation. This exercise should give the physician a good idea of how their documentation would fare in an audit or review. It would also give the physician insight into choosing a level of service based on the components outlined by these guidelines.

Let medical decision-making lead the way

The documentation guidelines recognize four levels of medical decision-making—straightforward, low complexity, moderate complexity, and high complexity. The level of medical decision-making is based on the following criteria:

- The number and severity of diagnoses and management options

- The amount/complexity of data obtained, reviewed, or analyzed

- The risk of significant complications, morbidity, or mortality

FIGURE 10.1	MEDICAL DECISION-MAKING		
A Problem type	**B** Amount of data to be ordered/ reviewed	**C** Risk of complications/ morbidity or mortality	**D** Type of decision-making
Minimal Limited Multiple Extensive	Minimal or none Limited Moderate Extensive	Minimal Low Moderate High	Straightforward Low Complexity Moderate Complexity High Complexity

Two of the three elements in the table below must be either met or exceeded to support a particular level of medical decision-making.

To arrive at a particular level of medical decision-making, two of the three areas above must be met or exceeded. For example, to support moderate complexity medical-decision making, the documentation must support, as a minimum, one of the following combinations from the table above.

Example 1	Example 2	Example 3
Multiple (Column A)	Multiple (Column A)	Moderate (Column B)
Moderate (Column B)	Moderate (Column C)	Moderate (Column C)

The **Figures 10.2–10.5** explain columns A–C in greater detail. Transfer the results regarding the number diagnoses and management options, amount and complexity of data, and the overall risk to the chart above and circle the transferred data. Draw a line down any column with two or three circles and circle the level of decision-making in that column, or draw a line down the column with the center circle and circle the level of decision-making in that column.

FIGURE
10.2

MEDICAL DECISION-MAKING

The mechanism used to determine a level of medical decision making is based on a point system that takes into account the number of diagnoses and management options, amount of data ordered or reviewed, and the risk of significant complications, morbidity, and/or mortality. Table A is used to determine the points associated with the number of diagnoses and problem types.

Table A			
Number of diagnoses and problem types			
Problem type		Points	Total
Minor/self limited Stable/improved/worsening	Maximum of 2 problems of this type	1	
Established problem Stable/improving		1	
Established problem Worsening/failing to change as expected		2	
New problem No additional workup planned	Maximum of 1 problem of this type	3	
New problem Additional workup planned		4	
			Total

	Points
FIGURE 10.3 TABLE B: AMOUNT OF DATA ORDERED/REVIEWED	

• Review/order of tests in CPT radiology section (nuclear medicine and all imaging except echocardiography and cardiac cath) (one or more tests ordered/reviewed = 1 point)   1

• Review/order of clinical lab tests (same scoring rule as above)   1

• Review/order of tests in CPT medicine section (EEG, EKG, Echocardiography, cardiac cath, non-invasive vascular studies, pulmonary function studies) (Same scoring rule as above)   1

• Discussion of test results with performing physician   1

• Independent review of image, tracing, or specimen   2

• Decision to obtain old records/obtain history from someone other than the patient   1

• Review and summarization of old records/history obtained from someone other than the patient   2

Total: _____

<table>
<tr><td colspan="4">FIGURE 10.4 — TABLE C: RISK OF SIGNIFICANT COMPLICATIONS, MORBIDITY, MORTALITY</td></tr>
</table>

Level of Risk	Presenting Problems	Diagnostic Procedures Ordered	Management Options
Minimal	• One self-limited or minor problem (e.g., cold, insect bite, tinea corporis)	• Lab tests requiring venipuncture • Chest x-rays • EKG/EEG • Urinalysis • KOH prep • Ultrasound, (echocardiography)	• Rest • Superficial Dressings • Gargles • Elastic bandages
Low	• Two or more self-limited or minor problems • One stable chronic illness, e.g., well controlled hypertension or non-insulin dependent diabetes, cataract, BPH • Acute uncomplicated illness or injury (e.g., cystitis, simple sprain, allergic rhinitis)	• Physiologic tests not under stress (e.g., pulmonary function tests) • Non-cardiovascular imaging studies with contrast (e.g., barium enema) • Superficial needle biopsies • Clinical lab tests requiring arterial puncture • Skin biopsies	• Over the counter drugs • Minor surgery with no identified risk factors • Physical therapy • Occupational therapy • IV fluids without additives
Moderate	• One or more chronic illnesses with mild exacerbation, progression, or side effect of treatment • Two or more stable chronic illnesses • Undiagnosed new problem with uncertain prognosis (e.g., lump in breast) • Acute illness with systemic symptoms (e.g., pnuemonitis, colitis, pyelonephritis) • Acute complicated injury (e.g., head injury with brief loss of consciousness)	• Physiologic tests under stress (e.g., cardiac stress test, fetal contraction stress test) • Diagnostic endoscopies with no identified risk factors • Deep needle or incisional biopsy • Cardiovascular imaging studies with contrast & no identified risk factors (e.g., arteriogram, cardiac catheterization) • Obtain fluid from body cavity (e.g., lumbar puncture, culdocentesis)	• Minor surgery with identified risk factors • Elective major surgery (e.g., open percutaneous, or endoscopic) • Prescription drug management • Therapeutic nuclear medicine • IV fluids with additives • Closed treatment of fracture or dislocation without manipulation
High	• One or more chronic illnesses with severe exacerbation, progression or side effect of treatment • Acute or chronic illnesses or injuries that may pose a threat to life or bodily function (e.g., multiple trauma, acute MI, pulmonary embolus, severe respiratory distress, progressive severe rheumatoid arthritis, psychiatric illness with potential threat to self or others, peritonitis, acute renal failure) • Abrupt change in neurologic status (e.g., sensory loss, seizure)	• Cardiovascular imaging studies with contrast with identified risk factors • Cardiac electrophysiological tests • Diagnostic endoscopies with identified risk factors • Discography	• Elective major surgery (e.g., open percutaneous or endoscopic) • Emergency major surgery (e.g., open, percutaneous or endoscopic) • Parenteral controlled substances • Drug therapy requiring intensive monitoring for toxicity • Decision not to resuscitate or to de-escalate care because of poor prognosis

Use the highest level of risk in any category to determine the overall level of risk

FIGURE
10.5

TABLE D: TYPE OF DECISION-MAKING

Problem type score	0 or 1	2	3	4
Data score	0 or 1	2	3	4
Overall risk	Minimal	Low	Moderate	High
Decision-making	Straightforward	Low complexity	Moderate complexity	High complexity

History

This chart outlines the history elements—history of the present illness, review of systems, and past family and social history. The instructions for finding the level of history are contained in the gray boxes located under the history chart.

A problem-focused history includes
- a brief history of the present illness

An expanded problem-focused history includes
- a brief history of the present illness
- a problem pertinent system review

A detailed history includes
- an extended history of the present illness
- an extended system review
- a pertinent past, family, and social history

FIGURE *10.6*	MEDICAL DECISION MAKING		

History			
HPI	ROS	PFSH	History type
• Location • Timing • Quality • Context • Severity • Modifying factors • Duration • Associated signs and symptoms	• Constitutional (fever,weight loss) • Eyes • Ears, nose, mouth, throat • Cardiovascular • Respiratory • Gastrointestinal • Genitourinary • Musculoskeletal • Integumentary • Neurologic • Psychiatric • Endocrine • Hematologic, lymphatic • Allergic, immunologic	**Past History** The patient's experience with illnesses, operations, injuries and treatments. **Family History** A review of medical events in the patient's family, including diseases which may be hereditary or place the patient at risk. **Social History** An age appropriate review of past and current activities (e.g., marital status, living arrangements, drugs, alcohol, tobacco, sexual history)	
Brief = 1-3 elements	None	None	Problem-focused
Brief	Problem pertinent = 1 system reviewed	None	Expanded problem-focused
Extended	Extended = 2-9 systems reviewed	Pertinent = at least 1 item from 1 of the 3 history areas	Detailed
Extended = 4 or more elements of the status of at least 3 chronic or inactive conditions	Complete = 10 or more systems reviewed	Complete = 1 item from 2 areas (established OV/emergency) 1 item from each of the 3 areas	Comprehensive
Using a previously documented encounter, determine the level of HPI, ROS, and PFSH documented. Circle the level of each on the chart.			
If a row has 3 elements circled, draw a line across that row to the right and circle that history, OR			
If no row has all the elements circled, find the circle(s) furthest to the top and draw a line across that row to the right and circle the type of history			

A comprehensive history includes

- an extended history of the present illness
- a complete system review
- a complete past, family, and social history

Exam

A Medicare carrier uses the exam guidelines most beneficial to the physician when performing an audit—typically the 1995 exam guidelines. Therefore, they are included in the chart below. For the 1997 general multi-system exam guidelines, go to *www.cms.hhs.gov/medicare*.

Medicare auditors are instructed to give credit from the set of guidelines (1995 or 1997) that is most beneficial to the physician. Many reviewers find the 1995 guidelines most beneficial to physicians who treat a broad spectrum of patients. However, the 1997 guidelines may be more beneficial to specialists.

Using a previously documented encounter, hospitalists should determine the number of body areas and organ systems examined and include vitals taken by practitioners and reviewed by the physician. All other exam elements must be personally performed by the physician to be counted. To qualify as a comprehensive exam, only organ systems must be counted. Body areas examined may not be included in the count. For example, an exam of the neck could not be counted as an organ system. However, if nodes in more than one area of the body were examined, it could be counted as the lymphatic system.

FIGURE
10.7

1995 EXAM E/M DOCUMENTATION GUIDELINES

Systems	Body areas	Exam type

• Constitutional
• Eyes
• Ears, nose, mouth, throat
• Cardiovascular
• Respiratory
• Gastrointestinal
• Genitourinary
• Musculoskeletal
• Integumentary
• Neurological
• Psychiatric
• Endocrine
• Hematologic/lymphatic
• Allergic/immunologic
	• Head, including
	  the face
	• Neck
	• Chest, including
	  breasts and axillae
	• Abdomen
	• Genitalia, groin, buttocks
	• Back, including spine
	• Each extremity
		Problem-focused
		Limited exam of system or area
		of present illness
		
		Expanded problem-focused
		(2-4 systems/body areas)
		Limited exam of system or area
		of present illness and related systems
		
		Detailed
		(5-7 body areas/organ systems)
		Extended exam of system and area of pre-
		sent illness and other necessary systems
		
		Comprehensive
		Complete exam of 8 or more organ systems

It is important to note that "complete exam," as described in the 1995 guidelines under the comprehensive level, has not been defined. This is precisely why the 1997 guidelines were developed. The intent was to give physicians a better idea of what the Centers for Medicare & Medicaid Services (CMS—the Health Care Financing Administration at that time) and the American Medical Association considered a complete exam of the various organ systems.

Documentation requirements

Initial encounters must meet the criteria for all three key components of history, exam, and medical decision-making. The following tables outline the types of history, exam, and medical-decision making the physician must document to support a particular code or level of service.

Subsequent encounters must meet the criteria for two of the three key components of history, exam, and medical decision-making. The physician should ensure that medical decision-making is one of the two required components met. The medical decision-making component gives the best picture of medical necessity—the need for a particular service, or service level. Insurers audit not only to determine that the documentation supported the level of service billed, but to also determine whether the level of service provided was necessary to treat the patient.

Medicare critical care guidelines

A clarification of Medicare's policy regarding payment for and medical review of critical care services is warranted. To reliably and consistently determine that delivery of critical care services is medically necessary, the following medical review criteria must be met in addition to the CPT definitions:

- Clinical condition criterion—a high probability of sudden, clinically significant, or life-threatening deterioration in the patient's condition that requires the highest level of physician preparedness to urgently intervene.

FIGURE 10.8	MEDICAL DECISION MAKING		

Code type	History	Exam	Medical decision-making
IP-Initial			
99221	Detailed or comprehensive	Detailed or comprehensive	Straightforward or low
99222	Comprehensive	Comprehensive	Moderate
99223	Comprehensive	Comprehensive	High
Admit/discharge same date			
99234	Detailed or comprehensive	Detailed or comprehensive	Straightforward or low
99235	Comprehensive	Comprehensive	Moderate
99236	Comprehensive	Comprehensive	High
Observation			
99218	Detailed or comprehensive	Detailed or comprehensive	Straightforward or low
99219	Comprehensive	Comprehensive	Moderate
99220	Comprehensive	Comprehensive	High
Emergency			
99281	Problem-focused	Problem-focused	Straightforward
99282	Expanded problem-focused	Expanded problem-focused	Low complexity
99283	Expanded problem-focused	Expanded problem-focused	Moderate complexity
99284	Detailed	Detailed	Moderate complexity
99285	Comprehensive	Comprehensive	High Complexity
IP-Consult			
99251	Problem-focused	Problem-focused	Straightforward
99252	Expanded problem-focused	Expanded problem-focused	Straightforward
99253	Detailed	Detailed	Low
99254	Comprehensive	Comprehensive	Moderate
99255	Comprehensive	Comprehensive	High

- Treatment criterion—critical care services require direct personal management by the physician. They are life- and organ-supporting interventions that require frequent, personal assessment and manipulation by the physician. Withdrawal or failure to initiate these interventions on an urgent basis would likely result in sudden, clinically significant or life-threatening deterioration in the patient's condition.

FIGURE
10.9

MEDICAL NECESSITY DECISION-MAKING

Code Type IP-subsequent	History	Exam	Medical Decision-making
99231	Detailed or comprehensive	Detailed or comprehensive	Straightforward or low
99232	Comprehensive	Comprehensive	Moderate
99233	Comprehensive	Comprehensive	High

FIGURE
10.10

DISCHARGE CODES: THESE CODES ARE TIME-BASED

Code type	Observation Discharge	Inpatient Discharge
99217	• Document all discharge services provided to the patient on this date	
99238	• Document all discharge services provided to the patient on this date	
99239	• Document all discharge services provided to the patient on this date and document time spend in providing discharge services. This must be physician time and may not include nursing time. To support this code the physician must have spent at least 31 minutes providing discharge services to the patient.	

Remember, not all medical care provided to a critically ill patient meets the definition of a critical care service. The physician service must be medically necessary and meet the definition of critical care services to be covered.

For example, a dermatologist treating a rash on an intensive care unit patient—on a ventilator and nitroglycerine drip managed by an intensivist—should not bill for critical care. Also remember that carriers may not automatically deny a claim if the patient's medical record indicates that a result or finding from a single test or procedure is "within normal limits," or indicates improvement in response to therapy. Carriers must look for additional indications in the medical record that all criteria (i.e., the CPT definition and medical review criteria) indicate that medical necessity and coverage are met. A patient with a designated status of "do not resuscitate" (e.g., organ donor) may qualify for critical care services when medical review criteria are met.

Full attention requirement for critical care

CPT 2000 eliminated the requirement for "constant attention" as a prerequisite for use of critical care codes. The new language states that CPT critical care codes 99291 and 99292 should be used to report the "total duration of time spent by a physician providing critical care services to a critically ill or critically injured patient, even if the time spent by the physician on that date is not continuous. For any given period of time spent providing critical care services, the physician must devote his or her full attention to the patient and, therefore, cannot provide services to any other patient during the same period of time."

Reporting physician time

CPT 2000 details the activities physicians count as critical care time. CPT 2000 requires a physician to document the time he or she spends with an individual patient in the patient's record. Physicians are permitted to report critical care time they spend engaged in work directly related to the individual patient's care, whether that time was spent at the patient's bedside or elsewhere on the floor or unit.

For example, the physician can report the time he or she spends on the unit reviewing test results or imaging studies, discussing the critically ill patient's care with other medical staff members, or documenting critical care services in the medical record as critical care. In addition, when the patient is unable or clinically incompetent to participate in discussions, the time the physician spends on the unit with family members or surrogate decision-makers obtaining a medical history, reviewing the patient's condition or prognosis, or discussing treatment or limitation(s) of treatment may also be reported as critical care of such conversations directly affect the medical decision-making.

CPT 2000 states that the "time spent in activities that occur outside of the unit or off the floor (e.g., telephone calls—whether taken at home, in the office, or elsewhere in the hospital) may not be reported as critical care since the physician is not immediately available to the patient. Time spent in activities that do not directly contribute to the treatment of the patient may not be reported as critical care, even if they are performed in the critical care unit (e.g., participation in administrative meetings or telephone calls to discuss other patients)."

Non-critically ill or injured patients in a critical care unit

CPT 2000 states that "services for a patient who is not critically ill but happens to be in a critical care unit are reported using other appropriate E/M codes," which means that the physician should not use critical care codes for a patient who receives medical care in a critical care, intensive care, or other specialized care unit unless the services meet the

- CPT definition of critical illness/injury

- CPT definition of critical care services

- medical review criteria

For example, patients who may not satisfy Medicare criteria for critical care payment include

- patients admitted to a critical care unit because no other hospital beds were available

- patients admitted to a critical care unit for close nursing observation/ frequent monitoring of vital signs

- patients admitted to a critical care unit because hospital rules require that certain treatments (e.g., insulin drips) are administered in the critical care unit

Physicians should report care of patients that does not meet all of the above criteria using the appropriate E/M codes (e.g., subsequent hospital visit codes 99231–99233, or inpatient consultation codes 99251–99255) depending on the level of service provided.

Ventilator management

The Medicare physician fee schedule final rule, published on December 10, 1993, prohibits payment for both an E/M service and ventilator management. The final rule states, "We will continue to recognize the ventilator management codes (CPT codes 94656, 94657, 94660, and 94662) as physician services payable under the physician fee schedule. Physicians will no longer be paid for ventilation management in addition to an E/M service, even if the E/M service is billed with CPT modifier -25."

Services bundled with critical care services

The following services, when performed on the same date the physician bills for critical care services, are included in the critical care service and should not separately reported:

- Interpretation of cardiac output measurements (CPT 93561, 93562)

- Chest x-rays (CPT 71010, 71015, 71020)

- Blood gases

- Blood draw for specimen (HCPCS G0001)

- Information data stored in computers—e.g., ECGs, blood pressures, hematologic data (CPT 99090)

- Gastric intubation (CPT 91105)

- Pulse oximetry (CPT 94760, 94762)
- Temporary transvenous pacing (CPT 92953)

- Ventilator management (CPT 94656, 94657, 94660, 94662)

- Vascular access procedures (CPT 36000, 36410, 36600)

- Family medical psychotherapy (CPT 90846)

Services that are not listed above may be reported separately. Remember, the physician should not include the time he or she spends performing services in addition to critical care services in the critical care time billed.

Services such as intubation and central line placement are considered procedures and require a distinct note in the medical record. However, the following services do not require modifiers when performed on the same date as other procedures and do not incur a multiple procedure payment reduction when billed on the same date as other procedures:

- **Intubation**

  Endotracheal, emergency procedure (31500). It may be billed in addition to critical care services.

- **Central line placement**

  Placement of central venous catheter (subclavian, jugular, or other vein) for central venous pressure, hyperalimentation, hemodialysis, or chemotherapy (36488), percutaneous, age two years or under (36489), percutaneous, over age two (36490), cut down, two years or under, and (36491) cut down, over two years. These codes may be billed on the same date as critical care services.

Use of a consultation code in conjunction with central line placement should be rare. Generally, physicians are asked to place the line rather than asked their opinion about placing the line. If a consultation on central line placement is billed, the documentation must clearly include the request for an opinion from the consulting physician, the particular conditions that warranted heightened concern for the patient's welfare if a central line were placed, and the consulting physician's response to the requesting physician.

Critical care services are time-based codes

Critical care codes are time-based services. The physician must document the time he or she spends providing critical care services to the patient.

FIGURE
10.11

CRITICAL CARE SERVICES ARE TIME-BASED CODES

Code type Critical care	
Less than 30 minutes	Use appropriate type and level of E/M code
30–74 minutes	99291 (1 unit of service)
75–104 minutes	99291 (1 unit) and 99292 (1 unit)
105–134 minutes	99291 (1 unit) and 99292 (2 units)
135–164 minutes	99291 (1 unit) and 99292 (3 units)
165–194 minutes	99291 (1 unit) and 99292 (4 units)
194 minutes and longer	99291 and 99292 as appropriate

- Critical care services provided to infants 31 days through 24 months are reported with pediatric critical care codes 99293 and 99294

- Critical care services provided to neonates (30 days of age or less) should be reported with neonatal critical care codes 99295 and 99296

Prolonged service codes

Physicians should use these codes when providing prolonged service involving direct patient contact beyond the typical time usually associated with the service. These codes are add-on codes and billed in addition to the appropriate level of E/M service. The physician must provide at least 31 minutes of face-to-face service beyond the typical service time to bill a prolonged service code. Medicare will only pay for the codes reflecting face-to-face services.

- **CPT codes 99356–99357—Prolonged inpatient physician service**

    99356: This service describes prolonged physician service in the inpatient setting requiring direct (face-to-face) patient contact beyond the usual service. This is an "add on" code and must be billed in addition to another E/M code. It cannot be billed alone. Physicians should bill the first 31–74 minutes of service beyond the typical time of the E/M code using this code. This could include services such as prolonged physiological monitoring or prolonged care of an acutely ill inpatient.

    99357—Physicians should use this code for each additional 30 minutes. Keep in mind that 99357 is an add-on code to 99356 and may not be billed alone.

    For example, a level two admission service is rendered, 99222, to a 65-year-old smoker with bronchitis who is in acute respiratory distress. The patient has complications (not qualifying as critical care) throughout the day. During the day and evening, the physician spends a total of 90 min-

utes face-to-face with the patient, including admission time. The physician should add the prolonged service code 99356 to the claim since
the typical time needed to care for 99222 is 50 minutes. However, the
physician spent an additional 40 minutes with the patient over the
course of the day. The service would be billed using codes, 99222 and
99356. The codes must be submitted on the same claim form, and the
documentation must clearly include the number of minutes spent providing services to the patient on that date.

FIGURE 10.12 — PROLONGED SERVICE CODES

Total duration of prolonged service	Code
Less than 30 minutes	Use appropriate type and level of E/M code
30–74 minutes	99356 (1 unit of service)
75–104 minutes	99356 (1 unit) and 99357 (1 unit)
105–134 minutes	99356 (1 unit) and 99357 (2 units)
135–164 minutes	99356 (1 unit) and 99357 (3 units)
165–194 minutes	99356 (1 unit) and 99357 (4 units)

Modifiers

A modifier is an indicator that alerts a payer that the service rendered some-how differs from the CPT description of the service, or falls outside the nor-mal processing or bundling edits used by insurers. Universal modifiers are generally two-digit numeric indicators. However, Medicare uses a number of two digit alpha modifiers in addition to the universal modifiers.

The following list in not all-inclusive. For more information, refer to the CPT book and contact the local Medicare carrier for a complete modifier listings.

- **24—Unrelated E/M service by the same physician during a post-operative period**
  The physician may need to indicate that an E/M service was performed during a postoperative period for a reason unrelated to the original procedure. The modifier is added to the E/M code.

- **25—Significant, separately identifiable E/M service by the same physician on the same day of the procedure or other service**
  This modifier indicates that the E/M service provided was unrelated to, or above and beyond the other service provided, or beyond the typical services associated with a procedure.

- **55—Postoperative management only**
  The physician should use this modifier when he or she performed the postoperative management and a different physician (different group or specialty) performed the surgical service. This often occurs when an

itinerant surgeon is involved. The modifier is added to the same procedure code used by the surgeon. The local Medicare carrier should have
specific billing instructions for the use of this modifier.

• **76—Repeat procedure by the same physician**
This modifier indicates that a procedure or service was repeated subsequent to the original procedure or service (identical services). The modifier is added to the second service billed.

• **77—Repeat procedure by another physician**
This modifier is used to indicate that a procedure or service was repeated subsequent to the original procedure or service performed by another physician. It is added to the procedure or service code.

Diagnosis coding basics

The primary reason for the encounter should be coded as the primary diagnosis. Remember, additional diagnosis codes should also be listed. Many processing delays are caused by missing or improper diagnosis codes. Therefore,
the physician must ensure that he or she is billing ICD-9 codes correctly.
Failure to communicate the necessary level of detail regarding diagnosis may
cause incorrect coding and unnecessary claim denials.

The interpreting physician should code the ICD-9 code that provides the
highest degree of accuracy and completeness for the diagnosis resulting from
a test, or for the signs and symptoms that prompted him or her to order the
test.

There has been some confusion in the past about the meaning of "highest degree of specificity," and "reporting the correct number of digits." In the context of ICD-9 coding, the "highest degree of specificity" refers to assigning the most precise ICD-9 code that most fully explains the narrative description of the symptom or diagnosis.

For example, if a sputum specimen is sent to a pathologist and the pathologist confirms growth of "streptococcus, type B," which is indicated in the patient's medical record, the pathologist should report a primary diagnosis as 482.32 (pneumonia due to streptococcus, group B). However, if the pathologist is unable to specify the organism, the pathologist should report the primary diagnosis as 486 (pneumonia, organism unspecified).

To report the correct number of digits when using ICD-9, refer to the following instructions:

- ICD-9 diagnosis codes are composed of codes with three, four, or five digits. Codes with three digits are included in ICD-9 as the heading of a category of codes that may be further subdivided by the use of fourth or fifth digits to provide greater specificity. Assign three-digit codes only if there are no four-digit codes within that code category. Assign four-digit codes only if there is no fifth-digit subclassification for that category, and assign the fifth-digit subclassification code for those categories where it exists.

  For example, a patient is referred to a physician with a diagnosis of diabetes mellitus. However, there is no indication that the patient has diabetic complications or that the diabetes is out of control. It would be incorrect to assign code 250 since all codes in this series have five digits. Reporting only three digits of a code that has five digits would be inappropriate. The physician must add two more digits to make the code accurate and complete. Because the type (adult onset/juvenile) of diabetes is not specified, and there is no indication that the patient has a complication or that the diabetes is out of control, the correct ICD-9 code is 250.00. The fourth and fifth digits of the code vary depending on the specific condition of the patient.

Basics of coding diagnostic tests

If the physician has confirmed a diagnosis based on the results of a diagnostic test, the physician interpreting the test should code that diagnosis. The signs and symptoms that prompted the physician to order the test may be reported as additional diagnoses if they are not fully explained or related to the confirmed diagnosis.

For example, a chest x-ray reveals a primary lung cancer in the left lower lobe. The interpreting physician should report the ICD-9 code as 162.5 for malignancy of the left "lower lobe, bronchus or lung", not the code for a malignancy of "other parts of bronchus or lung" (162.8) or the code for "bronchus and lung unspecified" (162.9). The signs or symptoms leading to the test may also be coded.

If the diagnostic test did not provide a diagnosis or was normal, the interpreting physician should code the sign(s) or symptom(s) that prompted the treating physician to order the study. Further, if the results of the diagnostic test are normal or nondiagnostic, and the referring physician records a diagnosis preceded by words that indicate uncertainty (e.g., probable, suspected, questionable, rule out, or working), then the interpreting physician should not code the referring diagnosis. Rather, the interpreting physician should report the sign(s) or symptom(s) that prompted the study. Diagnoses labeled as uncertain are considered by the *ICD-9 Coding Guidelines* as unconfirmed and should not be reported. This is consistent with the requirement to code the diagnosis to the highest degree of certainty.

Incidental findings should never be listed as primary diagnoses. If reported, incidental findings may be reported as secondary diagnoses by the physician interpreting the diagnostic test. In addition, unrelated and coexisting conditions or diagnoses may be reported as additional diagnoses by the physician interpreting the diagnostic test.

When a diagnostic test is ordered in the absence of signs/symptoms or other evidence of illness or injury, the physician interpreting the diagnostic test should report the reason for the test (e.g., screening) as the primary ICD-9 diagnosis code. The results of the test, if reported, may be recorded as additional diagnoses.

For the latest ICD-9 coding guidelines, go to *www.cdc.gov/nchs*, choose "ICD Information."

Helpful Web sites

Physicians can find helpful coding information on the Internet. However, it is a good idea to stick to official sites when the accuracy of coding and billing is at stake. Physicians should call their state's Medicare and Medicaid or Public Aid carrier for information on their Web sites and list servs.

www.cdc.gov/nchs	Information about diagnosis coding
www.cms.hhs/gov	National coverage determinations
	Local medical review policies
	Documentation guidelines for E/M services
www.oig.hhs.gov/	Office of Inspector General's *Work Plan*
	Safe harbor regulations
	Fraud alerts
	Compliance guidance
	Self-disclosure information
www.aha.org	The American Hospital Association
www.hhs.gov/ocr	HIPAA information
www.cms.hhs.gov/medlearn	CMS-sponsored coding and fraud abuse training
www.ahima.org	American Health Information Management Association
www.aapc.com	American Academy of Professional Coders